Handbook of
Pigmentary
Disorders
for Practitioners

Handbook of
Pigmentary
Disorders
for Practitioners

Editors

Kabir Sardana MD, DNB, MNAMS
Professor
Department of Dermatology and STDs
PGIMER, Dr Ram Manohar Lohia Hospital
New Delhi

Pooja Arora Mrig MD, DNB, MNAMS
Associate Professor
Department of Dermatology and STDs
PGIMER, Dr Ram Manohar Lohia Hospital
New Delhi

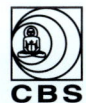

CBS

CBS Publishers & Distributors Pvt Ltd

New Delhi • Bengaluru • Chennai • Kochi • Kolkata • Mumbai
Hyderabad • Jharkhand • Nagpur • Patna • Pune • Uttarakhand

Handbook of
Pigmentary Disorders
for Practitioners

ISBN: 978-93-88108-97-3

Copyright © Editors and Publisher

First Edition: 2019
Reprint: 2021

Published by Satish Kumar Jain and produced by Varun Jain for

CBS Publishers & Distributors Pvt Ltd
4819/XI Prahlad Street, 24 Ansari Road, Daryaganj, New Delhi 110 002, India.
Ph: 011-23289259, 23266861, 23266867   Fax: 011-23243014   Website: www.cbspd.com
                                                                e-mail: delhi@cbspd.com; cbspubs@airtelmail.in
Corporate Office: 204 FIE, Industrial Area, Patparganj, Delhi 110 092
Ph: 011-4934 4934   Fax: 011-4934 4935   e-mail: publishing@cbspd.com; publicity@cbspd.com

Branches

- **Bengaluru:** Seema House, 2975, 17th Cross, K.R. Road,
  Banasankari 2nd Stage, Bengaluru 560 070, Karnataka
  Ph: +91-80-26771678/79   Fax: +91-80-26771680   e-mail: bangalore@cbspd.com
- **Chennai:** 7, Subbaraya Street, Shenoy Nagar, Chennai 600 030, Tamil Nadu
  Ph: +91-44-26680620, 26681266   Fax: +91-44-42032115   e-mail: chennai@cbspd.com
- **Kochi:** 42/1325, 1326, Power House Road, Opp KSEB, Power House, Ernakulam 682 018, Kochi, Kerala, India
  Ph: +91-484-4059061-67   Fax: +91-484-4059065   e-mail: kochi@cbspd.com
- **Kolkata:** 6/B, Ground Floor, Rameswar Shaw Road, Kolkata-700 014, West Bengal
  Ph: +91-33-22891126, 22891127, 22891128   e-mail: kolkata@cbspd.com
- **Mumbai:** PWD Shed, Gala No. 25/26, Ramchandra Bhatt Marg, Next to JJ Hospital, Gate No. 2,
  Opposite Union Bank of India, Noorbaug, Mumbai 400 009, Maharashtra, India
  Ph: +91-22-24902340/41/42   Fax: +91-22-24902342   e-mail: mumbai@cbspd.com

Representatives

• **Hyderabad**	0-9885175004	• **Jharkhand**	0-9811541605	• **Nagpur**	0-9421945513	• **Patna**	0-9334159340
• **Pune**	0-9623451994	• **Uttarakhand**	0-9716462459				

Printed at Nutech Print Services, Faridabad, India

to

---

*my patients for always inspiring me to keep learning and
having faith in me
and
to all my teachers for instilling knowledge and
providing guidance*

Pooja Arora Mrig

ॐ ईशा वास्यमिदँ सर्वं यत्किञ्च जगत्यांजगत् ।
तेनत्यक्तेनभुञ्जीथामागृधः कस्यस्विद्धनम् ॥१॥

*It is said that when Mahatam Gandhi was asked to
define joy in three words he said*
"Renunciation is Joy"

*Here he meant not to stop working for material gains, but
understanding the transitory nature of external embellishments.
If money itself brought joy, most wealthy people would
not be unhappy. Which is largely untrue.
In fact as Raman Maharishi has said*

*"The most peaceful time is when you sleep,
when you have no external wealth and when you are
detached from outside influences, hence wealth
does not really get you peace"*

*Coming back to the statement of Mahatama Gandhi, it is said that
"If all the Upanishads and all the other scriptures happened all of
a sudden to be reduced to ashes, and if only the first verse in the
Ishopanishad were left in the memory of the Hindus,
Hinduism would live forever"*

ॐ ईशा वास्यमिदँ सर्वं यत्किञ्च जगत्यांजगत् ।

*The Lord is enshrined in the hearts of all.
The Lord is also enshrined in all that pervades the Universe.
The Lord is the supreme Reality.*

तेनत्यक्तेनभुञ्जीथामागृधः कस्यस्विद्धनम् ॥१॥

*Rejoice in him through renunciation.
Covet nothing. Specially not others, wealth.
As All belongs to the Lord.*

Preface

"You aren't going to change the pigment of your skin...but you will find the pigment of your skin...will not be a hindrance".

Nivelle Goddard

Pigmentary disorders are one of the most common conditions encountered in dermatology practice. However, patients usually approach the general practitioners for these. Hence it is important to have basic knowledge of the common conditions so that the patient can be treated or referred accordingly. Sometimes the treatment can have more harmful effects than the underlying condition. And here lies the importance of initial treatment. The decision to treat or to refer should be made wisely by the doctor.

Most importantly, in Indian skin, the disorders take on a different hue and thus the Western books do not correctly reflect our skin.

We have divided the conditions into disorders of hypopigmentation and hyperpigmentation. We have tried to provide tables and photographs to make the text easier to understand. Chapters on Non-Melanin Pigmentation and Pigmented Skin Tumors have been added. We have discussed in detail the various aspects of treatment like topical and systemic therapy for hyperpigmentation and phototherapy for vitiligo.

Misuse of topical steroids is rampant these days which calls for the need of appraising the practitioners regarding appropriate use of topical steroids. This has been discussed in the chapter on Rational Use of Triple Combination Creams. The appendix outlines the classification and use of corticosteroids in dermatology.

We would especially like to thank Ms Nandita Das, the renowned actress who is associated with the 'Dark Is Beautiful' campaign, for her special contribution to this edition. She has expressed her views and concerns regarding the obsession with fairness and how it is destroying the self-esteem of millions of people, especially young girls.

A big thanks to the fabulous team at CBS Publishers & Distributors, Mr YN Arjuna Senior Vice-President—Publishing, Editorial and Publicity, and their team, Mrs Ritu Chawla Assistant General Manager—Production, Mr Vikrant Sharma and Mr Ram Murti. CBS is one of the few publishers who have invested in an advanced preproduction software that matches the quality of print before its out. This has been possible due to the ingenuity of Mr SK Jain CMD, Mr Varun Jain Director, and Mr SK Verma. It's a rare publisher who takes out a digital print for its authors before the book is out.

We hope the book serves the purpose for which it has been taken out and provides first-hand knowledge about pigmentary disorders.

Hope the readers are benefitted by it.

Happy Reading!

Kabir Sardana
Pooja Arora Mrig
Editors

Contributors

Aastha Gupta MD
Senior Resident
Dermatology
Dr RML Hospital and PGIMER
New Delhi

Arijit Coondoo MD
Professor
Department of Dermatology
KPC Medical College and Hospital
1F, Raja SC Malik Road
Kolkata

Gauri Vats MD
Senior Resident
Dermatology
Dr RML Hospital and PGIMER
New Delhi

Kabir Sardana MD, DNB, MNAMS
Professor
Dermatology
Dr RML Hospital and PGIMER
New Delhi

Manu Sehrawat MD
Ex-Senior Resident
Dermatology
Dr RML Hospital and PGIMER
New Delhi

Nandita Das
Actress, Director

Niharika Dixit MD
Senior Resident
Dermatology
Dr RML Hospital and PGIMER
New Delhi

Pooja Arora Mrig MD, DNB, MNAMS
Associate Professor
Dermatology
Dr RML Hospital and PGIMER
New Delhi

Contents

Basics and Introduction

Kabir Sardana, Pooja Arora Mrig

BASICS

This overview of pigmentary disorders is based on three fundamental concepts which are elucidated in the following pages. We will first focus on the role of melanocytes in the color of the skin. This is followed by an overview of various types of colors that can be visualized for numerous different skin diosrders without specifically being related to the melanocyte. At the end, we give an overview of the common pigmentation disorders both hyper and hypo.

Needless to say, it must be appreciated that no amount of manipulation by fairness creams can alter the basic nature of the skin in Indians nor can it affect in any way the melanocytes. This message should be conveyed to patients at the outset.

MELANOCYTES AND COLOR

Melanin, synthesized by melanocytes, provides some defence against ultraviolet radiation (UVR) as well as gives color to skin and hair. Skin color and ease of tanning are important determinants of the risk of skin cancer.

- **Melanocytes** are dendritic cells that migrate from the neural crest to the epidermis and hair follicles in the third month of fetal development.
- Melanocytes are interspersed amongst the basal keratinocytes in the epidermis. Melanocyte stem cells are found in the bulge region of hair follicles from where they migrate to the hair bulb.
- Melanocytes synthesize both brown/black eumelanin and red/yellow pheomelanin from tyrosine.
- Melanin is passed in packages (melanosomes) along dendritic processes into keratinocytes (Fig. 1.1) where melanosomes sit in a cap or 'parasol' over the upper sun-exposed side of the keratinocyte nucleus. Each melanocyte links to a number of keratinocytes, forming an epidermal melanin unit. Melanin provides protection by absorbing visible light and UVR.
- UVR induces tanning by stimulating oxidation of pre-existing melanin, by triggering the synthesis of new melanin, and by changing the distribution of melanosomes.
- Melanin is the main determinant of the color of skin and hair. The color depends on the number, size, and distribution of melanosomes within keratinocytes and

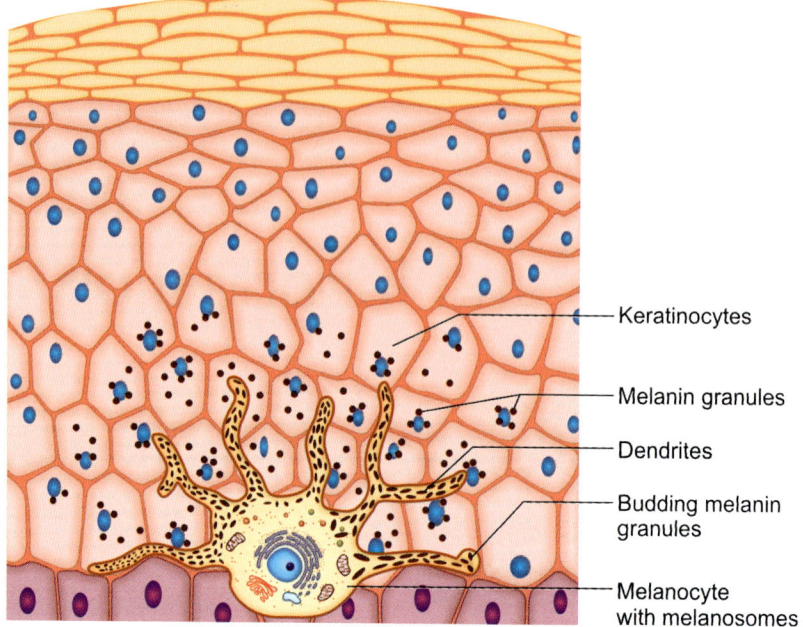

Fig. 1.1: An artist's depiction of the epidermis with the melanocyte which has dendritic processes that help in dispersing melanin to the keratinocytes

the type of melanin, rather than the number of melanocytes. Darkly pigmented skin has similar numbers of melanocytes as lightly pigmented skin, but more and slightly differently packaged melanin (melanosomes) within keratinocytes.

- The melanosomes in white skin are small and tend to be aggregated within the keratinocyte whereas in darker skin melanosomes are larger and distributed as singlets.

- Skin color is not uniform. Normal variation in pigment also called pigmentary demarcation lines must be differentiated from acquired pigmentation (Box 1.1). Dorsal skin surfaces are more pigmented

Box 1.1: Pigmentary demarcation lines (Voigt-Futcher lines)

Type A	Vertical line on the lateral aspect of the upper arm that may extend into the pectoral region (commonest).
Type B	Curved line on back of the thigh (posteromedial) that extends from the perineum to the popliteal fossa and occasionally the ankle.
Type C	Vertical or curved hypopigmented band on the mid-chest (contains two parallel lines).
Type D	Vertical line on the posteromedial area of the spine.
Type E	Bilateral hypopigmented streaks, bands, or patches on the upper chest in the zone between the mid-third of the clavicle and the periareolar skin.
Facial patterns, which appear around puberty, have been described in the Indian subpopulation:	
Type F	V-shaped hyperpigmented lines between the malar prominence and the temple.
Type G	W-shaped hyperpigmented lines between the malar prominence and the temple.
Type H	Linear bands of hyperpigmentation from the angle of the mouth to the lateral aspects of the chin.

than ventral surfaces. Lines of demarcation between darker dorsal and paler ventral surfaces are apparent in about 20% of people with dark skin. The lines, which are symmetrical and bilateral, are present from infancy and have no clinical significance.

• Darkly pigmented skin has better epidermal barrier function than lightly pigmented skin.

INTRODUCTION

COLOR AND SKIN DISORDERS

Most skin disorders have a distinctive color to them. Though we will largely discuss disorders with alteration in pigment cells (melanocytes), it is a good idea to give an overview of the various colors that can be seen in skin disorders. These are listed in Table 1.1. Disorders of melanin pigmentation can be divided into hypermelanosis and hypomelanosis. Hypermelanosis is characterized by increased amount of melanin in the skin. Excess melanin in epidermis gives a brownish hyperpigmentation whereas in the dermis it produces a blue or slate-gray appearance. Hypomelanosis is characterized by a lack of pigment in the skin that leads to white or lighter skin as compared to the normal color. Depigmentation refers to loss of pre-existing pigment from the skin. The commonly used term 'leukoderma' denotes white skin that can be congenital or acquired.

Table 1.1: Overview of causes of various colored lesions in dermatology			
Color		Common causes	
	Endogenous		Exogenous
Red/purple	Erythrocytes Inflammation Vessels	Hemangioma (Fig. 1.2)	Tattoo
Black	Melanin Inflammation Vessel occlusion Necrosis	Vessel necrosis (Fig. 1.3)	Tattoo Poison Ivy Tick
Blue	Melanin Vessels	Venous malformation (Fig. 1.4)	Drug Heavy metals Tattoo pigment
Yellow	Lipid CT disease Deposition Keratin	Xanthoma (Fig. 1.5a to c)	Drug
Brown	Melanin Hemosiderin Celullar proliferation (dermatofibroma)	Melasma (Fig. 1.6)	Drug
White	Decreased melanin Vasospasm Deposition (calcium) Keratin Scar	Scar (Fig. 1.7)	Tattoo

CT: Connective tissue

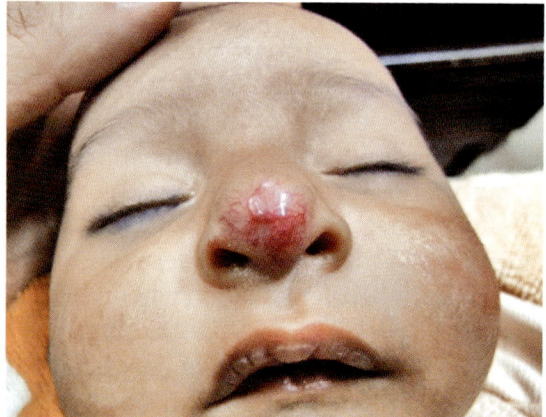

Fig. 1.2: Red nodule: Hemangioma

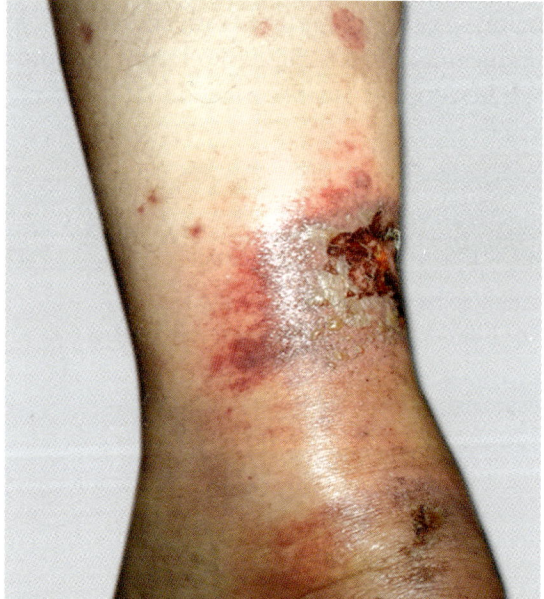

Fig. 1.3: Vessel necrosis in a case of occlusion with vasculitis

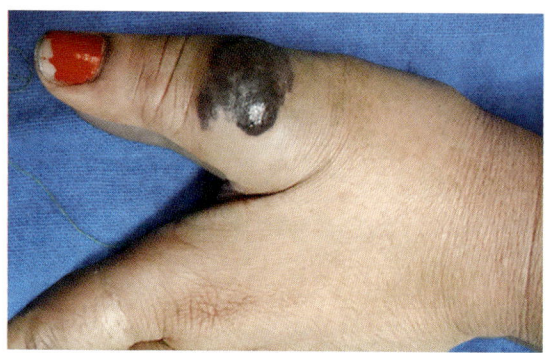

Fig. 1.4: Venous malformation

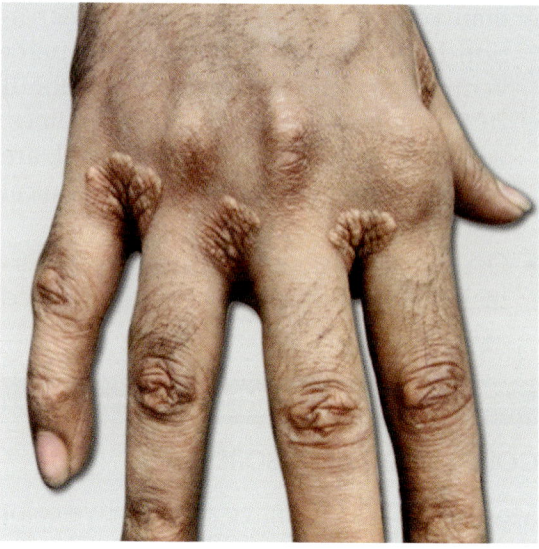

Fig. 1.5a: Striate xanthoma (type III hyperlipoproteine-mia)

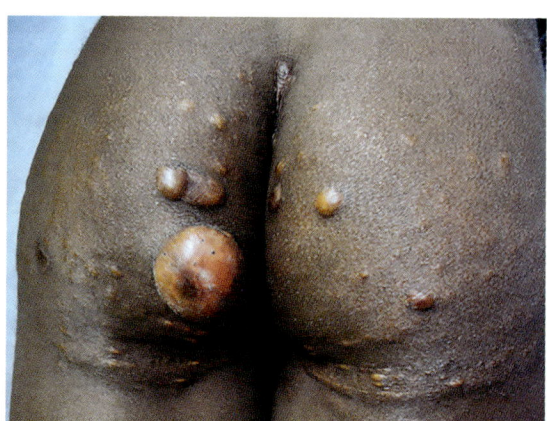

Fig. 1.5b: Tuberous xanthoma

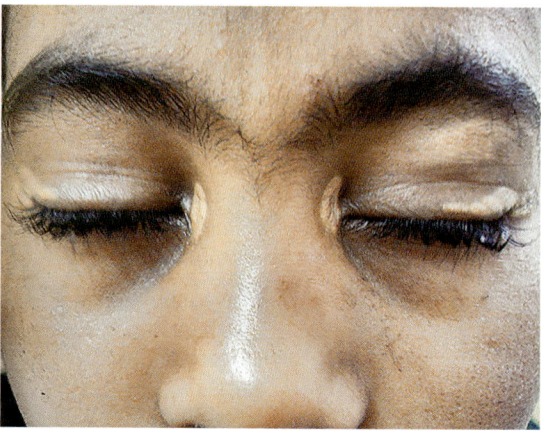

Fig. 1.5c: Xanthelasma

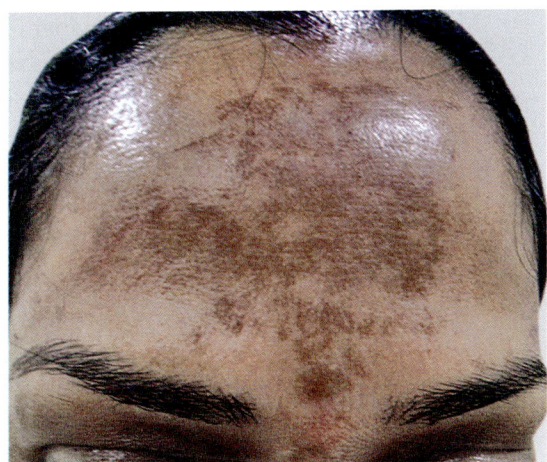

Fig. 1.6: Melasma

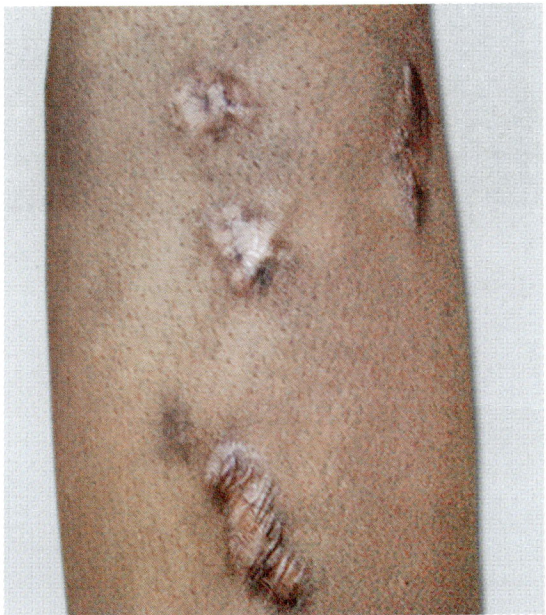

Fig. 1.7: Scar following traumatic injury

Change in Skin Color (Pigment Cell)

The commonest cause of change in color is due to a previous inflammation. This is known as post-inflammatory hyperpigmentation. Though we will be largely restricting ourselves to the change in melanin and melanocytes, it is important to take an overview of the various causes. The details of common disorders will follow in subsequent Chapters.

Acquired Hyperpigmentation

Strictly speaking, hyperpigmentation means brown skin, but this list encompasses colors ranging from brown to blue or gray.

a. **Common**
- Normal racial variation or sun tan.
- *Stasis dermatitis*: The pigment is a mixture of melanin and hemosiderin.
- *Melasma* (*usually facial*): Brown color caused by melanin (Fig. 1.6).
- Post-inflammatory hyperpigmentation, particularly in dark skin.
  Common after acne, lichenoid eruptions such as lichen planus (LP) or cutaneous lupus erythematosus (LE) and contact dermatitis (Fig. 1.8a). Lichenoid eruptions subside with a grayish tinge as the pigment is deep in the dermis (Fig. 1.8b).
- 10% of normal people have one or two café au lait spots/macules (CALM) (Fig. 1.9).
- *Erythema ab igne*: Repeated local heating of the skin from a hot water bottle or fire causes localized fixed reticulate pigmentation.
- *Phytophotodermatitis*: Linear streaks of brown pigmentation are preceded by erythema and sometimes blisters.

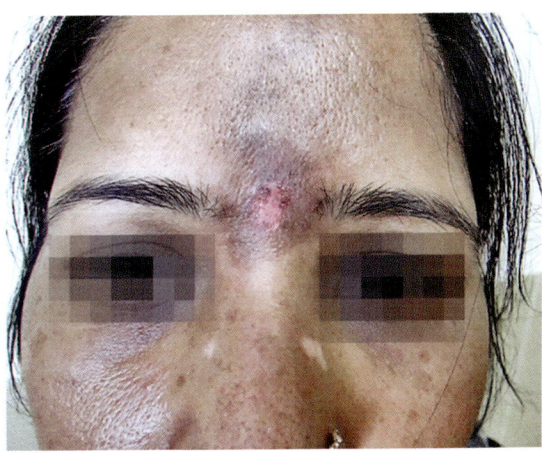

Fig. 1.8a: Contact dermatitis—due to the allergy to the sticking chemical of bindi

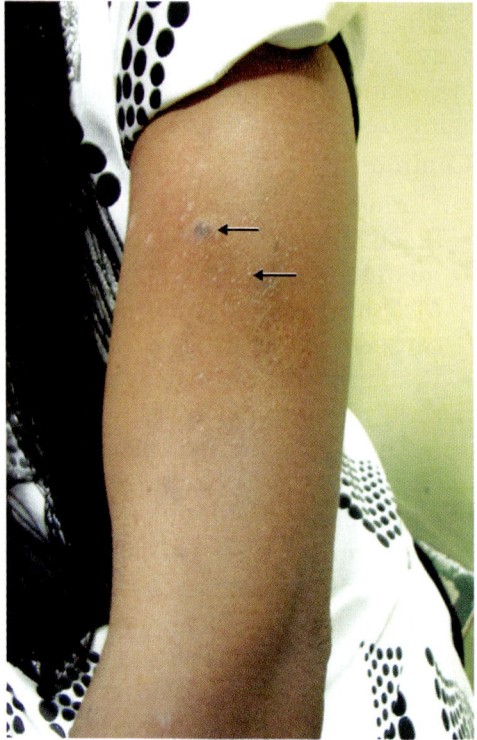

Fig. 1.8b: Lichenoid eruption

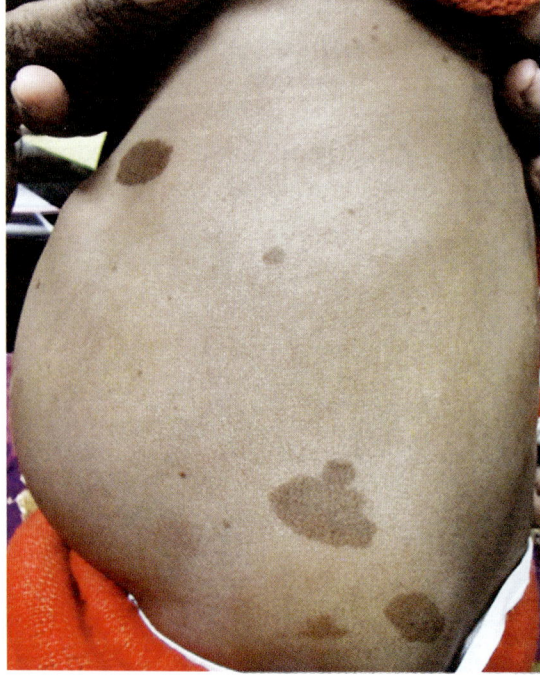

Fig. 1.9: CALM. Here the patient has multiple CALM. It is advisable to look for a systemic cause

- *Dermatitis neglecta:* Occasionally, patients avoid touching a patch of skin. The unwashed skin builds up brown scale.
- Drugs, including minocycline, antimalarials (Fig. 1.10), amiodarone, and heavy metals, may give the skin a bluish grey tinge.
- *Amyloidosis:* Rippled pigmentation (Fig. 1.11).

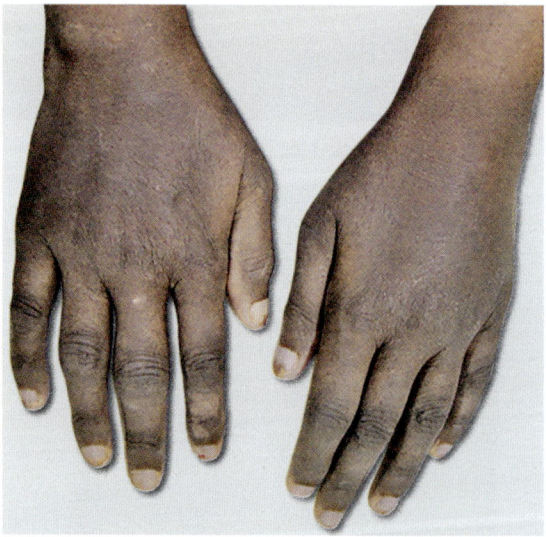

Fig. 1.10: Drug-induced pigmentation: This patient was on HCQS (hydroxychloroquine sulfate) for 6 months

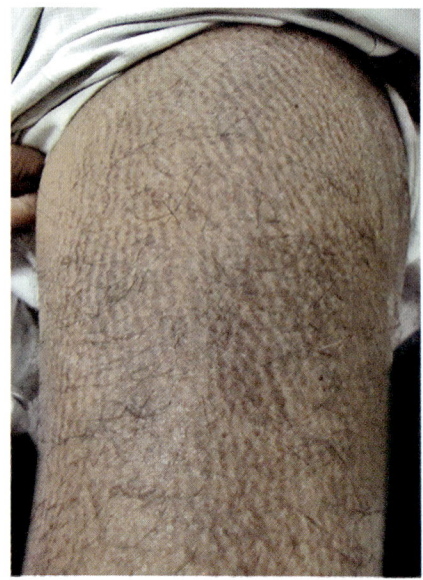

Fig. 1.11: Amyloidosis: Rippled pigmentation

b. **Less common**
- Neuropathic itch or chronic rubbing.
- Malabsorption, pellagra (Fig. 1.12).
- Cutaneous systemic sclerosis and sclerodermoid chronic graft versus host disease (GVHD). The skin is thickened, often with perifollicular hypopigmentation.

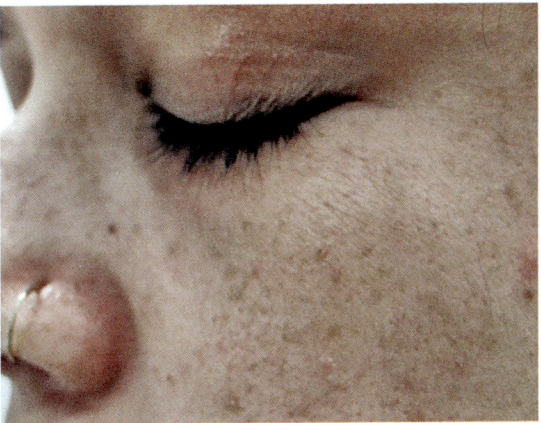

Fig. 1.13: Freckles in a fair-skinned patient

- Pseudo-ochronosis secondary to hydroquinone in skin-lightening creams (may also cause confetti-like loss of pigment). It is also called as exogenous ochronosis.
- Primary biliary cirrhosis, hemochromatosis.

c. **Rare**
- *Café au lait spots (CALM)*: Multiple CALMs are seen in neurofibromatosis, McCune-Albright syndrome, multiple mucosal neuromas syndrome.
- Widespread freckling (Fig. 1.13) in children may be associated with xeroderma pigmentosum (XP), multiple lentigines syndrome, Carney complex, and Peutz-Jeghers syndrome.
- *Generalized pigmentation:* Adrenal insufficiency, Nelson syndrome, ectopic adrenocorticotropic hormone (ACTH)—producing tumors, POEMS syndrome in plasma cell disorders.
- *Alkaptonuria:* Blue black pigment of helices of the ear and sclerae.

Hypopigmentation and Depigmentation

Hypopigmented skin: Loss of pigment is partial. The tone of the skin is creamy, rather than absolutely white. Depigmented skin is

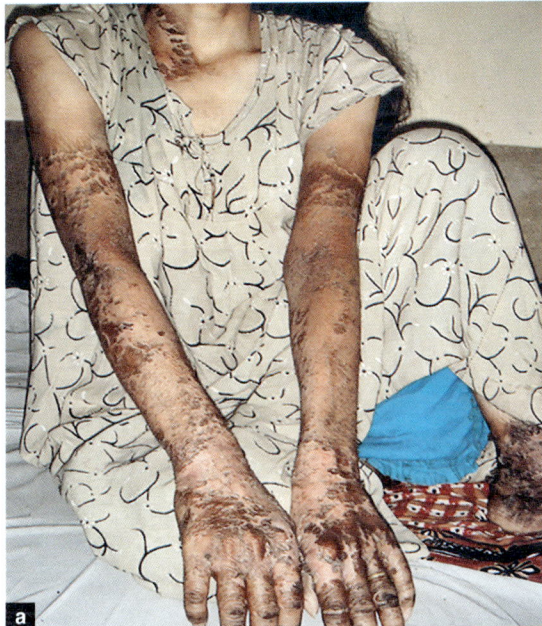

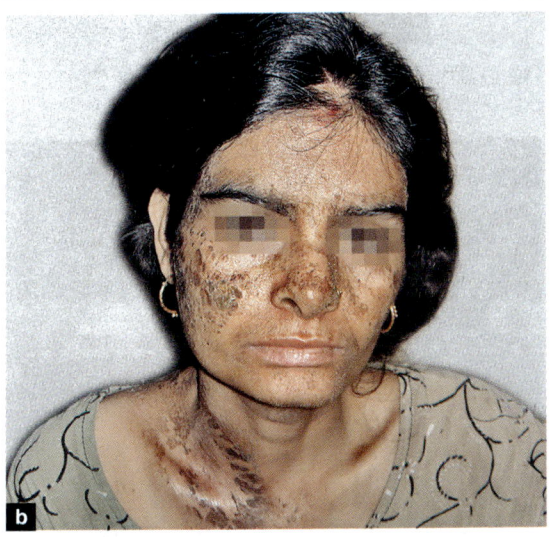

Fig. 1.12a and b: Pellagra: Scaly pigmented plaques on exposed sites

white and fluoresces bright white under Wood's light, e.g. vitiligo, though this is rarely required in our skin type.

a. **Common**

- *Pityriasis alba:* Hypopigmented cheeks in children. Subtle scale may be present (Fig. 1.14).
- *Pityriasis versicolor:* Scaly in the active phase, but macular post-inflammatory hypopigmentation may persist for months, until melanocytes are stimulated by sun exposure (Fig. 1.15).
- *Idiopathic guttate hypomelanosis:* Pale macules on sun-damaged forearms of adults.

- *Progressive macular hypomelanosis:* Common in young AfroCaribbean adults. Progressive symmetrical hypo-pigmentation in midline of the trunk.
- *Post-inflammatory hypopigmentation:* Most often in dark skin. Causes— psoriasis, discoid lupus erythematosus (DLE) (Fig. 1.16), sarcoidosis, leprosy, pinta, and kwashiorkor.
- *Vitiligo:* Smooth depigmented macules or patches (Fig. 1.17).
- *Halo nevus:* Seen in children or young adults, a ring of white skin appears around a melanocytic nevus. The brown 'mole' gradually turns pink and

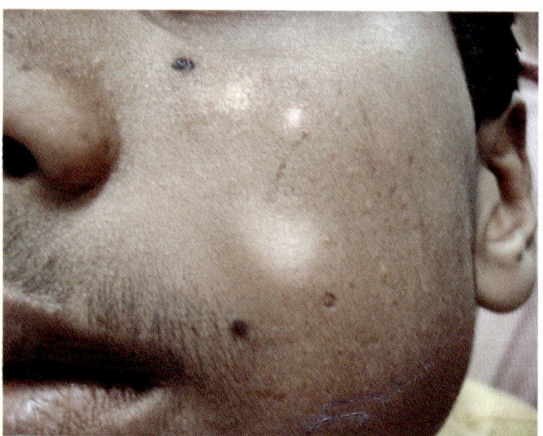

Fig. 1.14: Pityriasis alba

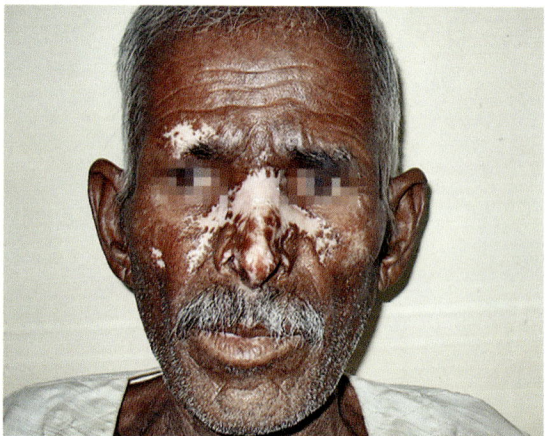

Fig. 1.16: DLE: Discoid plaques of DLE heal with pigmentary loss and can be mistaken for vitiligo

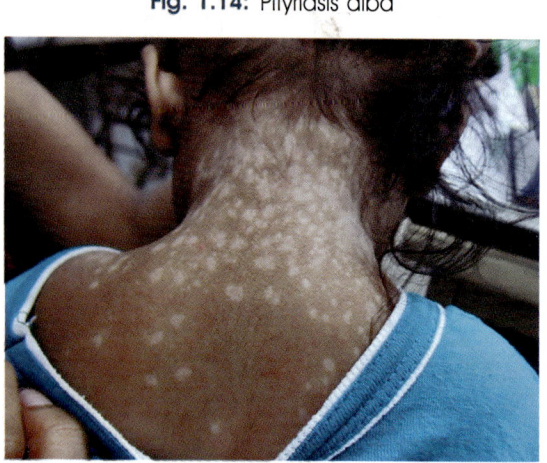

Fig. 1.15: Macular post-inflammatory hypopigmentation consequent to P versicolor

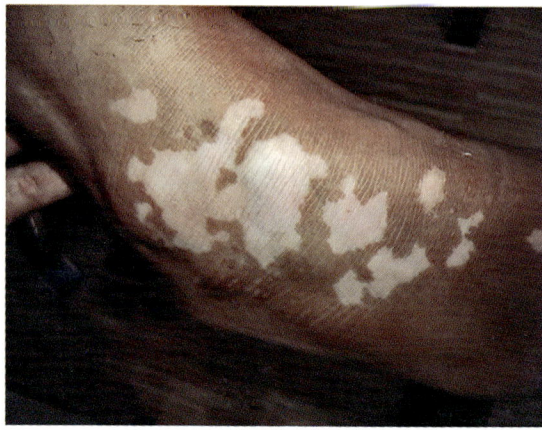

Fig. 1.17: Vitiligo

eventually disappears, leaving a depigmented macule (Fig. 1.18).

- Scars (may also be hyperpigmented).
- *Atrophie blanche:* Pale scar with a rim of telangiectasia. Seen over the leg in venous disease.
- *Post-injection:* Perilymphatic depigmentation consequent to injection of steroids within joints or ganglion is a common and reversible phenomenon (Fig. 1.19).

b. **Less common**
- Contact leukoderma after exposure to chemicals, e.g. aromatic or aliphatic

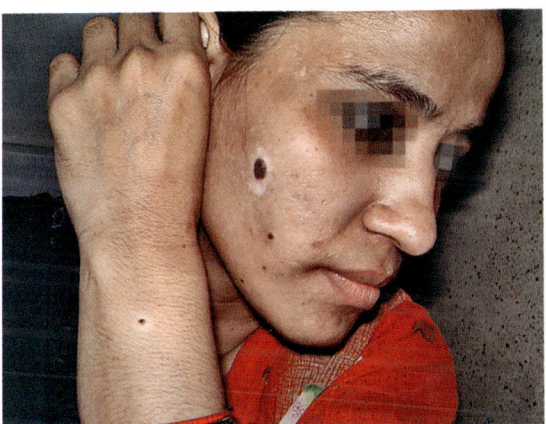

Fig. 1.18: Halo nevus

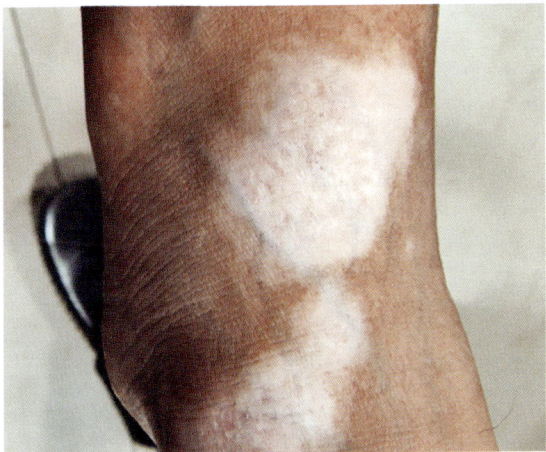

Fig. 1.19: Post-steroid pigmentary loss. Commonly seen due to extravasation of steroid while injecting intralesionally

derivatives of phenols or catechols, hydroquinone in skin-lightening creams, betel leaves, fentanyl patches.

- *Secondary syphilis:* Hypopigmented macules superimposed on hyperpigmented, reticulate patches (syphilitic leucomelanoderma) seen over neck, chest, and back. Usually occurs six months after primary disease.
- *Tuberous sclerosis:* Oval or confetti- like hypopigmentation.
- *Cutaneous lupus erythematosus (LE):* Hypo- and hyperpigmentation.
- *Morphea or cutaneous scleroderma:* Perifollicular hypopigmentation in thickened skin. May also be hyperpigmentation.
- Chronic GVHD (also hyperpigmentation).
- *Antiphospholipid syndrome:* Porcelain white scars with telangiectatic rim (like atrophie blanche).
- *Chronic arsenic ingestion:* 'Raindrop' hypopigmentation.
- *Extragenital lichen sclerosus:* Crinkly, shiny white papules with follicular plugging. Look for genital disease.
- *Nevus depigmentosus:* Localized hypopigmented skin with discrete, regular, or serrated margins. Stable appearance.
- *Nevus anemicus:* Jagged outline, caused by vasoconstriction
- Cutaneous T cell lymphoma (Fig. 1.20).

c. **Rare**
- Malignant atrophic papulosis (Degos disease). Erythematous papules evolve into porcelain white scars with a rim of telangiectasia. Linked to fatal vascular occlusion in the gastrointestinal tract (GIT) or central nervous system (CNS). Differentiate from antiphospholipid syndrome.
- *Pigmentary mosaicism:* Swirling hypopigmented patches (Fig. 1.21).

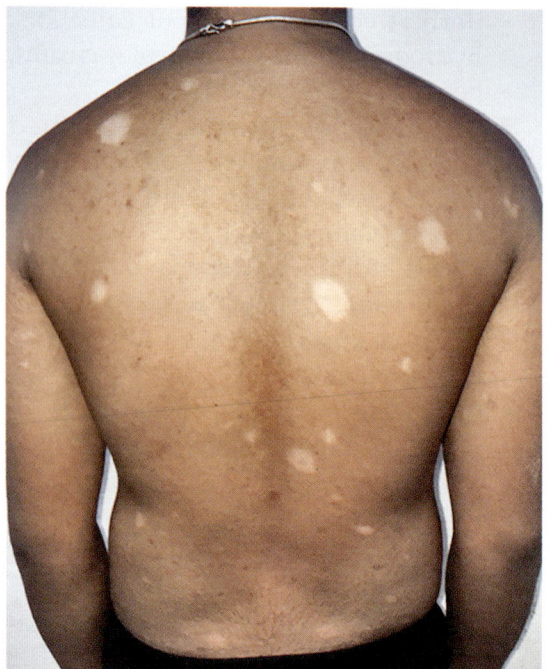

Fig. 1.20: A child with hypopigmented macules over the trunk. Biopsy showed changes suggestive of mycosis fungoides

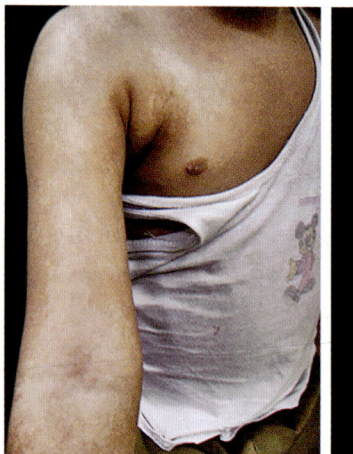
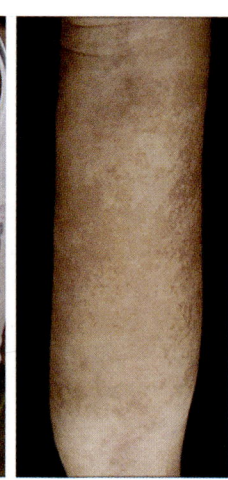

Fig. 1.21: Nevoid hypomelanosis

- Focal dermal hypoplasia of Goltz.
- *Albinism:* Total body depigmentation, light blue iris, nystagmus.
- Waardenburg syndrome (a form of piebaldism). Autosomal dominant (AD) inheritance. Symmetrical patches of hypopigmentation on the face, scalp, back, and proximal extremities, with a stripe of normal-colored skin down the center of the back. Also white forelock, neurosensory deafness, widening of the bridge of the nose, and hetero-chromia of the iris.
- *Incontinentia pigmenti:* Linear atrophic hypopigmented scars along Blaschko's

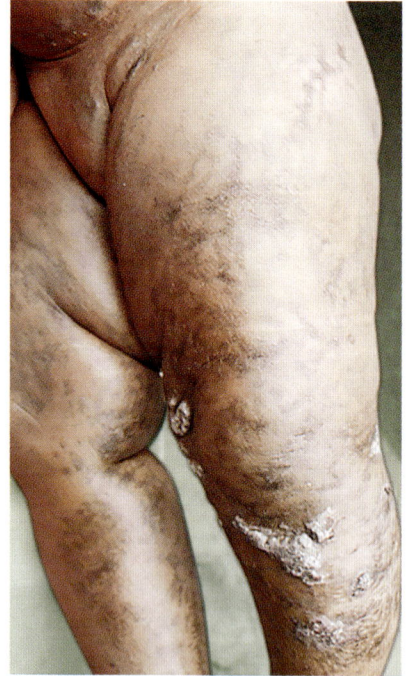

Fig. 1.22: Incontinentia pigmenti

lines that represent post-inflammatory scarring (Fig. 1.22).

Disorders of Hypopigmentation

Kabir Sardana, Pooja Arora Mrig

1. APPROACH TO HYPOMELANOTIC DISORDERS

Hypomelanotic disorders are skin conditions characterized by reduced melanin content of the lesional skin presenting as light-colored areas. **Depigmentation** refers to total absence of pigment from the lesions resulting clinically in milky white amelanotic patches. The disorders of hypomelanosis can be classified in various ways such as according to the age of onset, the extent of lesions and according to the underlying cause. For establishing a correct diagnosis, detailed history and clinical examination aided by biopsy and special investigations such as Wood's lamp examination, fungal scraping, etc. is often required. This chapter gives an overview of the common hypomelanotic disorders encountered in the dermatology practice.

The most common disorder presenting at birth with hypomelanotic lesion is *nevus depigmentosus*. It is a sporadic disorder presenting as hyopigmented macules with serrated margins on the trunk. The segmental form may pose diagnostic confusion with vitiligo but can be differentiated based on the age of onset and the morphology of the lesion. Other congenital causes of hypomelanosis include *piebaldism*, *albinism* and *leukoderma* seen in association with *tuberous sclerosis*.

Vitiligo is a common acquired pigmentary disorder presenting clinically with depigmented macules. The margins are typically scalloped and perifollicular pigment retention is characteristic of repigmenting patches. It may present in various forms such as, a localized macule (cutaneous/mucosal), segmental lesion, predominant acral involvement or diffuse cutaneous involvement. Associated findings include poliosis and scalp involvement. Histopathologically, the lesions show absence of melanin pigment. *Chemical associated leukoderma* is seen secondary to agents such as catechols, phenols, hydroquinone, etc. History of occupational exposure to such chemicals is important in clinching the diagnosis. The lesions are depigmented and begin at the site of contact with the chemical agent but may also involve unexposed sites causing diagnostic confusion with vitiligo.

Infections are a common cause of hypomelanotic lesions. The most common infection presenting with such features is *pityriasis versicolor*. It is caused by *Malassezia* species and presents with light-colored lesions over upper back and chest with overlying furfurous scaling that becomes more evident on scratching. The disorder is common in hot and humid climate and presents most commonly in young individuals. The diagnosis is aided by KOH examination of the scales which reveals spaghetti and meatball appearance of the hyphae and spores and also by characteristic fluorescence seen under Wood's lamp examination. Other infections associated with hypomelanotic lesions include leprosy, post-kala-azar dermal leishmaniasis, treponematosis and onchocerciasis.

Progressive macular hypomelanosis of the trunk is a pigmentary disorder that presents with nummular hypomelanotic nonscaly macules over the trunk. The pathogenesis of this disorder is unknown; however, a relation between the hypomelanotic macules and presence of *Propionibacterium acnes* has been hypothesized. Histological findings include reduction of pigment in the epidermis and occasional perifollicular infiltrate in the dermis. *Hypopigmented variant* of *mycosis fungoides* presents clinically with hyopigmented macules over the non-sun-exposed areas such as the trunk and the buttocks. The characteristic distribution of the lesions in an adult patient and histopathological evidence of epidermotropism of atypical lymphocytes in the epidermis establishes the diagnosis. Another malignancy which might present with alteration of pigment in the skin is melanoma. Three types of hypopigmentation are seen in association with *melanoma*. First is hypopigmentation appearing at sites of tumor regression, secondly pigmentary loss surrounding the tumor deposits and lastly hypomelanotic patches appearing at sites distinct to the site of primary tumor/metastasis.

Hypomelanosis as a consequence of *post-inflammatory* changes is a common entity encountered in dermatology practice. The most common disorder in this group is pityriasis alba. It presents with ill-defined hypomelanotic macules on the face. The etiology of this disorder is poorly understood. Proposed hypotheses include unprotected sun exposure, hot baths and cutaneous signs of atopy. Hypopigmentation is seen commonly in association with cutaneous disorders such as lupus erythematosus, scleroderma, lichen sclerosus, etc. Destruction of basal melanin-containing layer accounts for the depigmentation seen in these disorders, 'salt and pepper' appearance is classically seen in lesions of morphea and scleroderma. Lesions may clinically mimic repigmenting vitiligo with perifollicular pigment retention but induration can be felt on palpation which often aides in the diagnosis. The pathogenesis of lichen sclerosus includes genetic, autoimmune, hormonal, infectious, and local factors. Mechanisms responsible for leukoderma include decreased melanin production, reduced melanosome transfer and melanocyte loss. Sarcoidosis may also rarely present with hypopigmented lesions. Hypopigmentation is seen secondary to interface dermatitis. It is seen commonly in darkly pigmented individuals and lesions present on the extremities. Diascopy may aid in the diagnosis (yellowish tinge due to presence of granulomas).

Rare causes of generalized hypopigmentation include endocrine abnormalities such as hypothyroidism and hypogonadism and nutritional deficiency such as copper and selenium deficiency.

It is our opinion that a simple regional approach is a simple method of arriving at a diagnosis, even though not all skin disorders conform to this localization (Flowchart 2.1). The text that follows will detail the disorders within the flowchart in two broad categories of *common* and *rare* disorders.

Flowchart 2.1: Approach to diagnosis of hypopigmented disorders

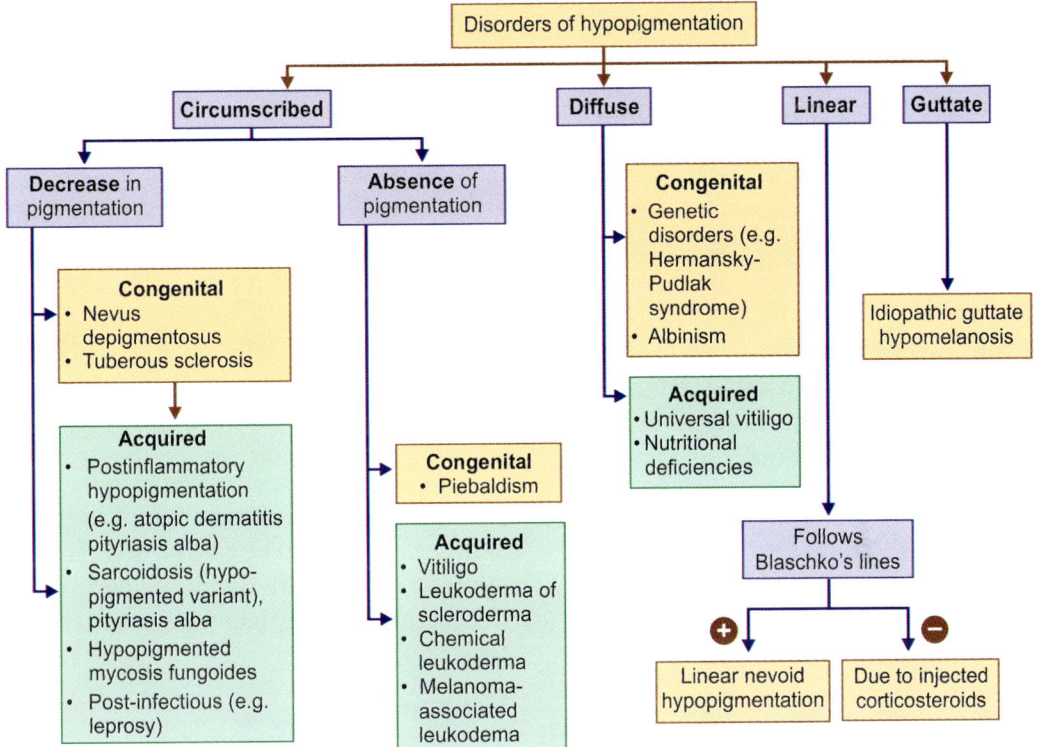

2. COMMON DISORDERS

PITYRIASIS ALBA

Incidence

This disease mainly affects children between the age of 3 and 16 years and is clinically obvious in dark-skinned individuals.

Pathogenesis

The exact cause is unknown, though it is formally recognized as postinflammatory hypomelanosis secondary to a low grade eczematous reaction. The following factors have been incriminated in its pathogenesis:

a. Excessive and unprotected sun exposure.
b. Frequent bathing with hot water, frequent washing of face with soap-based cleansers.
c. Cutaneous signs of atopy are associated with pityriasis alba.

Clinical Features

Pityriasis alba is characterized by multiple ill-defined hypopigmented macules and patches surmounted by fine, 'bran-like' (*pityron*, Greek for bran) scales (Fig. 2.1) and

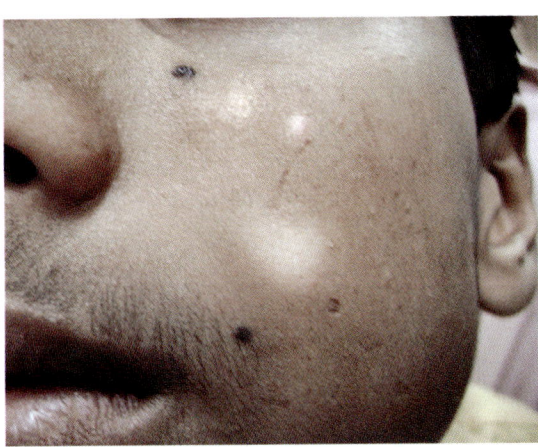

Fig. 2.1: A boy with dry skin and hypopigmented macules (pityriasis alba)

may persist for months or years before resolving spontaneously. The early lesion is a mildly erythematous, slightly scaling patch with an indistinct elevated margin. In children, the face is the most common area of involvement (Fig. 2.2a), although it can occur at any location and may have one to several lesions. The lesion/patch appears to get worse and flakier in winters, when the skin is dry. However, it is more noticeable in the summer when the pale skin stands out against a tan. It is usually asymptomatic, although an occasional patient may complain of mild itching. Patients or parents are most concerned about the appearance of the lesions.

Investigations

No specific laboratory test is available to establish the diagnosis. The KOH preparation is negative. The histological picture is nonspecific, showing slight hyperkeratosis, decreased pigmentation in the basal cell layer and a mild inflammatory reaction in the upper dermis (Fig. 2.2b).

Differential Diagnosis

Diagnosis is based on the clinical examination. A biopsy is rarely needed. In children, face is involved in one-third of cases of tinea

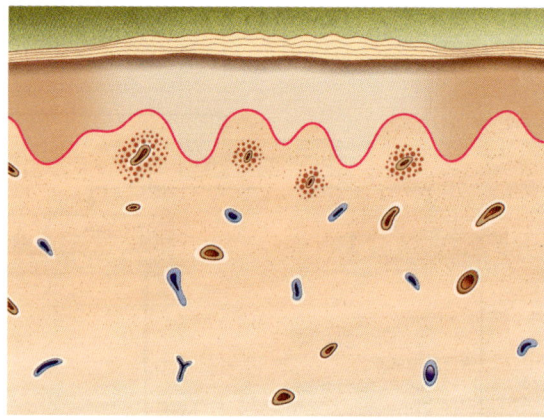

Fig. 2.2b: Epidermis—hyperkeratosis; decreased pigmentation. Dermis—mild inflammation around superficial blood vessels

versicolor. Thus, in doubtful cases, KOH skin scrapping can be performed. The white spots in vitiligo are distinguished by sharp demarcation, complete depigmentation and lack of scales.

Treatment

Treatment is not often necessary as spontaneous resolution occurs. Emollients can be used for the dry scaling, and 1% hydrocortisone cream is used for the inflammatory reaction.

Other steroids that can be used include desonide 0.05%, fluocinolone acetonide 0.01% (Table 2.1) and fluticasone propionate 0.05%.

Course and Complication

The patient must understand that repigmentation will be slow. In most patients, the disease resolves spontaneously, but this

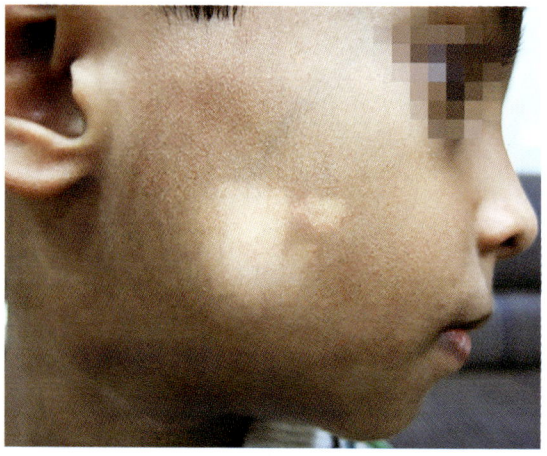

Fig. 2.2a: Pityriasis alba on the face

Table 2.1: Overview of the treatment for P alba		
	Medical management	
Topical	Emollients, mild corticosteroids, tacrolimus	
Oral	None	
Counseling	Patients should be reassured that this condition is not vitiligo	

takes months, and sometimes years. For affected children, the disease rarely persists into adulthood. The disease has no complications.

Bibliography

1. Jones JB. Eczema, Lichenification, Prurigo and Erythroderma. In: Burns T, Breathnach S, Cox N, Griffiths C, eds. Rook's Textbook of Dermatology, 8th edition. Oxford: Blackwell Science; 2010. Chapter 23, Pp. 23, 27–23.28.
2. Mollet I, Ongenae K, Naeyaert JM. Origin, clinical presentation, and diagnosis of hypomelanotic skin disorders. *Dermatol Clin.* 2007 Jul; 25(3): 363–71, ix.
3. Park HY, Yaar M. Biology of Melanocytes. In: Goldsmith LA, Katz SI, Gilchrest BA, Paller AS, Leffell DJ, Wolff K, eds. Fitzpatrick's Dermatology in General Medicine. Eighth edition, Chapter 72, Pp. 807–8.
4. Ruiz-Maldonado R. Hypomelanotic conditions of the newborn and infant. *Dermatol Clin.* 2007 Jul; 25(3):373–82, ix.

POST-INFLAMMATORY HYPOPIGMENTATION

Post-inflammatory hypomelanosis (PIH) represents a very common skin disorder that is more obvious in darkly pigmented or tanned individuals. A large number of dermatoses can lead to PIH (Table 2.2).

Clinical Features

Hypomelanosis usually follows or coexists with inflammatory lesions (Fig. 2.3a to c),

but occasionally, only hypopigmented lesions are seen, e.g. in sarcoidosis or mycosis fungoides.

Psoriasis

The epidermal hyperproliferation rate is increased in psoriasis. The melanin synthesis cannot keep pace with the increased rate leading to hypopigmentation (Fig. 2.3a and b). It can also occur due to application of potent topical steroids.

Eczema/Dermatitis

Eczema like seborrheic and atopic dermatitis can lead to hypopigmentation.

Table 2.2: Common disorders causing post-inflammatory hypopigmentation

1. Psoriasis
2. Seborrheic dermatitis
3. Atopic dermatitis
4. Lichen sclerosus
5. Lichen striatus
6. Lupus erythematosus
7. Leprosy
8. Syphilis

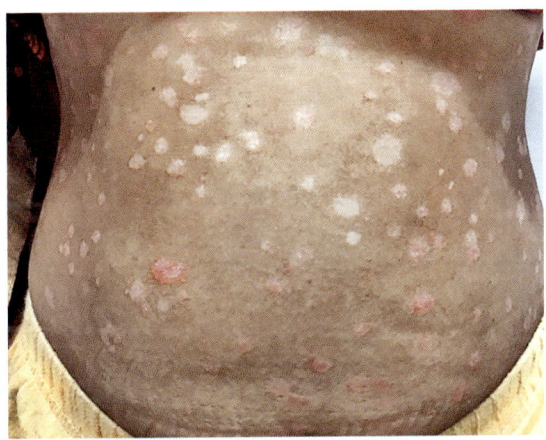

Fig. 2.3a: Lesions of psoriasis subsiding with hypopigmentation

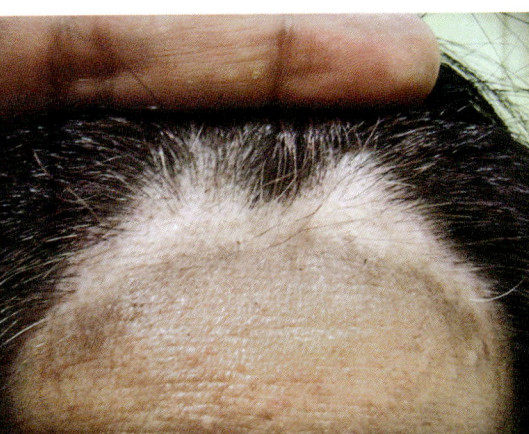

Fig. 2.3b: A case of psoriasis of the scalp healing with post-inflammatory hypopigmentation

Lichen Striatus

This condition is seen in children and is characterized by small pink or hypopigmented papules in the initial stage. These disappear spontaneously leaving linear hypopigmentation.

Lupus Erythematosus

In lupus erythematosus (LE), there is destruction of the basal layer containing melanocytes. A classical discoid lupus erythematosus (DLE) lesion is characterized by atrophy and depigmentation (Fig. 2.3c).

Scleroderma

Areas of depigmentation surrounded by hyperpigmentation may be seen in scleroderma. It is called 'salt and pepper' pigmentation.

Lichen Sclerosus

Lichen sclerosus (LS) is a chronic pruritic skin disorder that is more commonly seen in the anogenital region in post-menopausal females. It is characterized by milky white

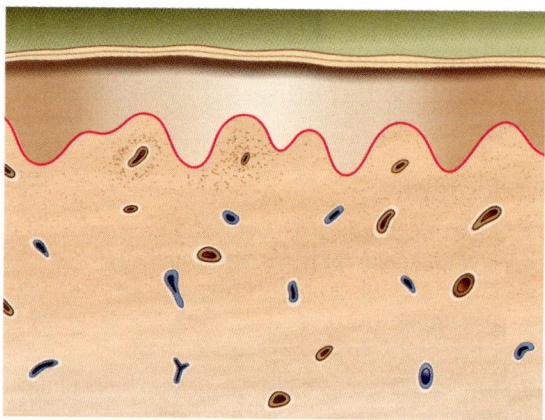

Fig. 2.3d: Epidermis is hypopigmented and dermis shows mild inflammation

atrophic papules with follicular plugging. The condition is severely itchy and can also lead to loss of labia minora.

Histology

The biopsy findings are non-specific but are depicted in Figure 2.3d.

Treatment

Once the underlying inflammatory disorder is effectively treated, the PIH usually resolves gradually.

a. Sun exposure or UVB phototherapy may be helpful. In amelanotic lesions with complete loss of melanocytes, epidermal or melanocyte grafting may be considered.

b. A very effective therapy is the use of a mild steroid (clobetasone butyrate 0.05%, desonide 0.05%, fluticasone propionate 0.05%) at night.

c. A vegetable oil (coconut oil) in the morning.

d. Tacrolimus can also be used in a similar fashion.

e. For patients with steroid phobia, topical tar 1–2% is a simple therapeutic intervention.

Bibliography

Pigmentation Disorders. In: Sardana K, Garg VK, Mahajan S, eds. Diagnosis and Management of Skin Diseases: An Evidence Base Approach, Wolters Kluwer, LWW 2012, 1st edition.

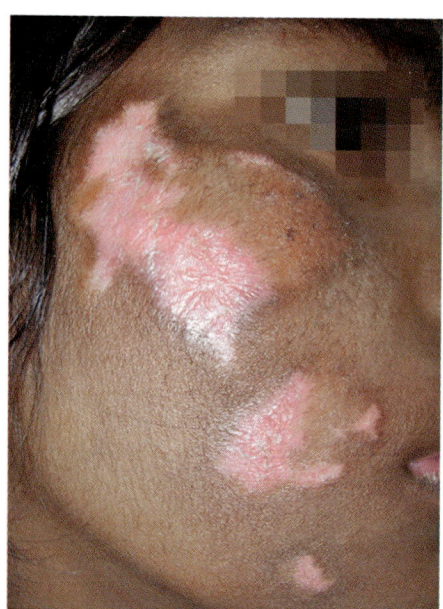

Fig. 2.3c: A case of discoid lupus with post-inflammatory depigmentation

VITILIGO

Vitiligo is an acquired disorder characterized by circumscribed depigmented macules and patches that result from a progressive loss of functional melanocytes. It is a cause of great stigma in India, though it has no major health consequences. Vitiligo is a multifactorial disorder related to both genetic and non-genetic factors. It is generally agreed that there is an absence of functional melanocytes in vitiligo skin.

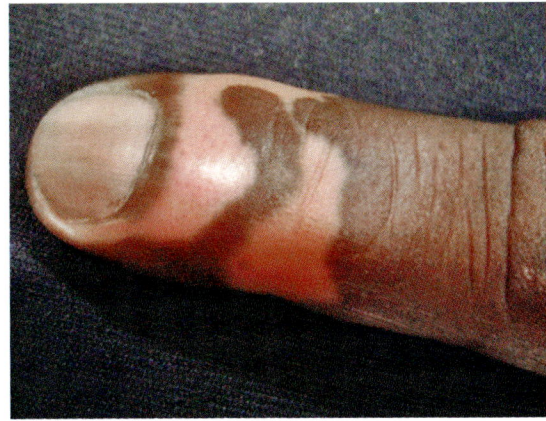

Fig. 2.4: A case of vitiligo on the digit, the erythema is consequent to phototherapy

Pathogenesis

Various theories have been suggested for the pathogenesis of vitiligo. Out of these, the "autoimmune" hypothesis is the most widely accepted and is backed by evidence. It is based on the fact that vitiligo is associated with various autoimmune diseases and there may be an underlying genetic susceptibility leading to these. Other factors involved in pathogenesis include dysregulation of innate and adaptive immune responses, increased oxidative stress, presence of antibodies to normal human melanocytes and role of cytotoxic T cells.

Clinical Features

The most common presentation of vitiligo is totally amelanotic (i.e. milk- or chalk-white) macules or patches surrounded by normal skin (Fig. 2.4). The borders are usually convex, as if the depigmenting process were "invading" the surrounding normally pigmented skin.

Lesions enlarge centrifugally overtime, though the rate may be slow or rapid.

Trichrome vitiligo features a hypopigmented zone between normal and totally depigmented skin (Fig. 2.5). The intermediate zone does not have a gradation of color from white to normal, but rather a fairly uniform hue. The number of melanocytes is also intermediate in this zone,

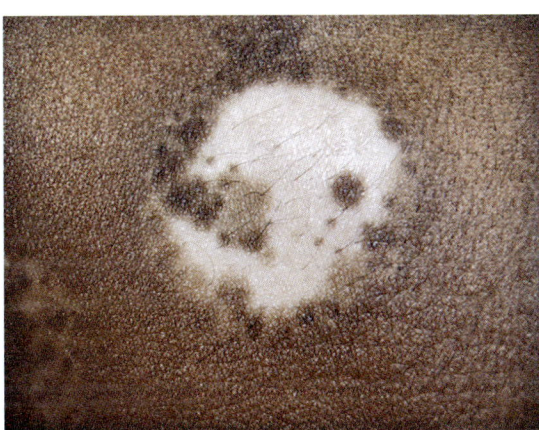

Fig. 2.5: A case of quadrichrome vitiligo. Apart from the three zones at the periphery (trichrome), there is perifollicular pigmentation. Note the presence of pigmented hair which is a good prognostic sign

suggesting slower centrifugal progression than in typical vitiligo. In *quadrichrome vitiligo*, a fourth darker color is present at sites of perifollicular repigmentation (Fig. 2.5). *Pentachrome vitiligo* with five shades of color—black, dark brown, medium brown (unaffected skin), tan and white—has also been described.

One of the manifestations of vitiligo is the isomorphic Koebner phenomenon (IKP), characterized by the development of vitiligo at the sites of trauma (e.g. a laceration, burn or abrasion).

Clinical Classification of Vitiligo

Multiple classification systems for vitiligo have been proposed, leading to confusing terminology. Two major forms are generally recognized:

1. The segmental form, which usually does not cross the midline; and
2. The non-segmental form, also called vitiligo vulgaris.

Another simpler classification is given in Box 2.1 and depicted in Fig. 2.6.

Box 2.1: Classification of vitiligo

Localized:
1. *Focal:* One or more macules in one area, but not clearly in a segmental distribution.
2. *Unilateral/segmental:* One or more macules involving a unilateral segment of the body; lesions usually stop abruptly at the midline (Fig. 2.7).
Generalized:
1. *Vulgaris:* Scattered patches in localized areas.
2. *Acrofacial:* Distal extremities and face (Fig. 2.8).
3. *Universal:* Generalized involvement.

Investigations

A search for other autoimmune conditions can be undertaken. This includes DM, SLE and autoimmune thyroiditis. They do not influence the therapy in any significant way. Wood's lamp can be used to aid diagnosis. Various clues to diagnosis of vitiligo include a family history of vitiligo, presence of Koebner's phenomenon or leukotrichia, and associated autoimmune diseases.

The biopsy can be performed and reveals absence of pigment (Fig. 2.8c).

Dermoscopy can be used to diagnose doubtful cases (Fig. 2.8d and e).

Diagnosis

Clinical in most cases.

Treatment

The aim of vitiligo treatment is repigmentation and stabilization of the depigmentation process. The choice of therapy depends on the extent, location, and activity of disease as well as the patient's age, skin type, and motivation to undergo treatment. In general,

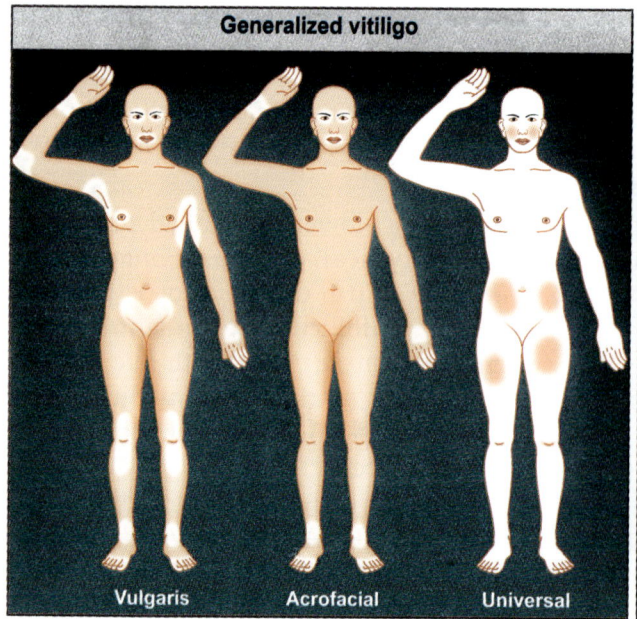
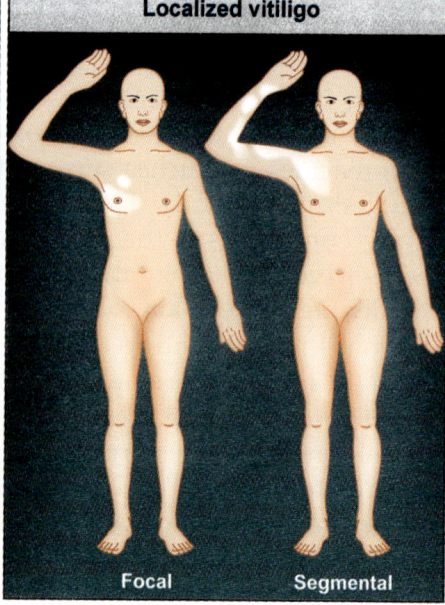

Fig. 2.6: A depiction of the types of vitiligo

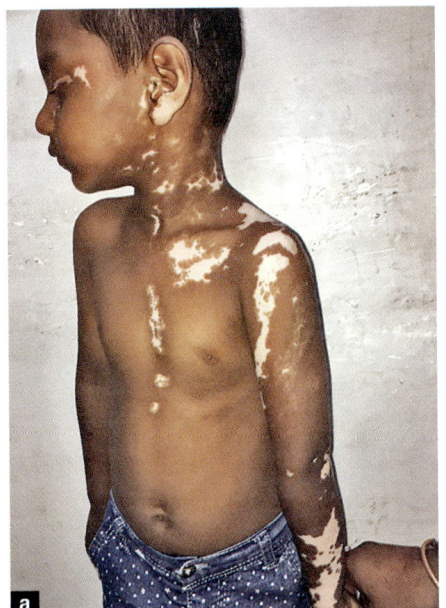

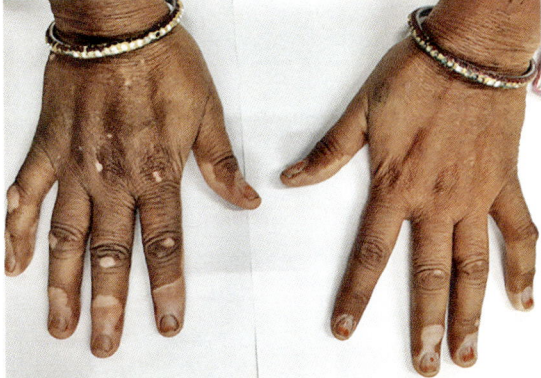

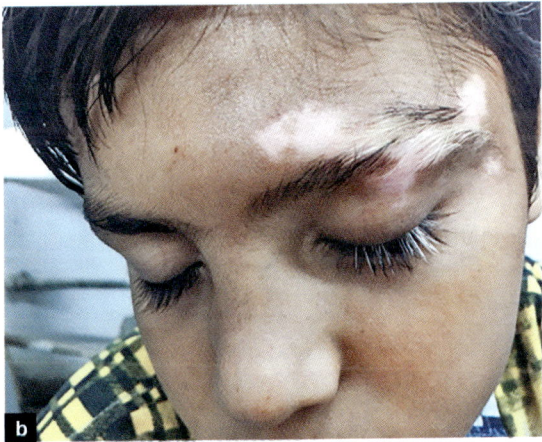

Fig. 2.7a and b: Segmental vitiligo in a young boy. Note the associated leukotrichia

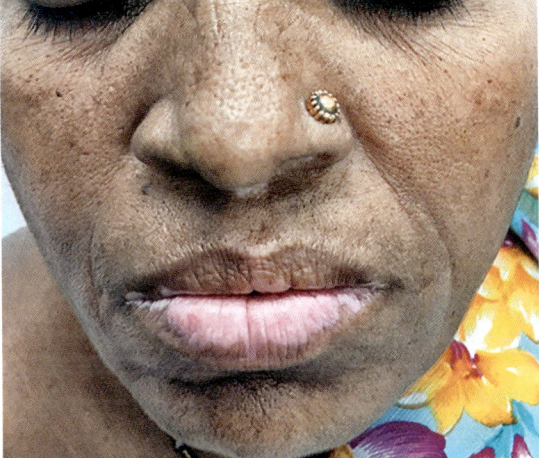

Fig. 2.8b: Lip tip vitiligo

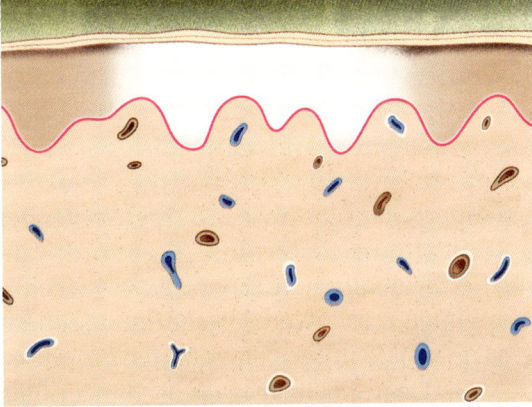

Fig. 2.8c: Epidermis—complete absence of pigment and melanocytes. Dermis—normal

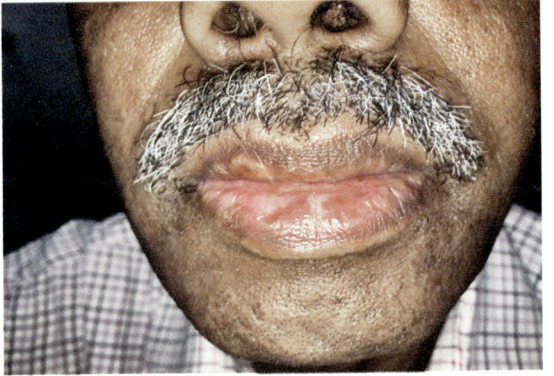

Fig. 2.8a: Lip vitiligo

a period of at least 2–3 months is required to determine whether a particular treatment is effective.

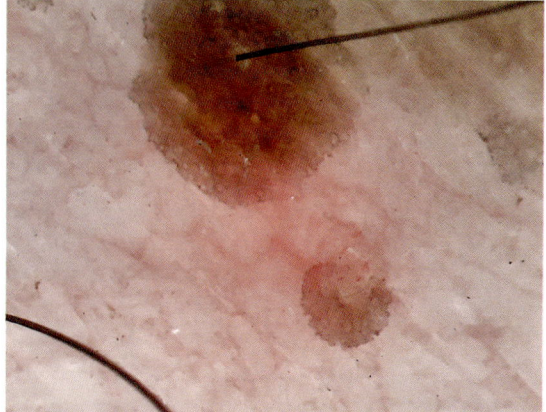

Fig. 2.8d: Vitiligo with perifollicular repigmentation

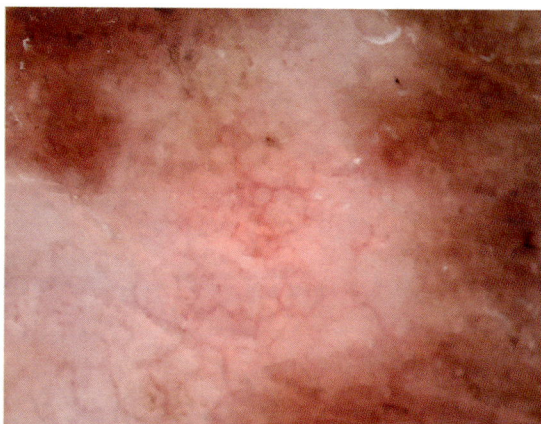

Fig. 2.8e: Vitiligo with increased vascularity due to steroid

The areas of the body that typically have the best response to medical therapy are the face, neck, mid-extremities, and trunk (Figs 2.9 to 2.11), while the distal extremities and lips are the most resistant to treatment (Fig. 2.4). Repigmentation usually appears in a perifollicular pattern and/or from the periphery of the lesions. When the hairs within an area of vitiligo are depigmented, the former pattern is not observed.

Medical Therapy

Most primary care clinicians can use topical treatments initially.

1. **Corticosteroids:** This is administered in vitiligo affecting <20% of the body surface area and can achieve >75% repigmentation with either class 1 (superpotent) or class 2–3 (high-potency) topical corticosteroids. To avoid side effects, an alternate day or twice/weekly regimen is followed. Discontinue, if there is no visible improvement after 2 months.

   Oral steroids have been used in a pulse form, but should be used only for cases with documented instability of disease. Though a common practice is to give betamethasone (Betnesol) twice a week, a safer alternative is to administer a short acting steroid to avoid side effects. An

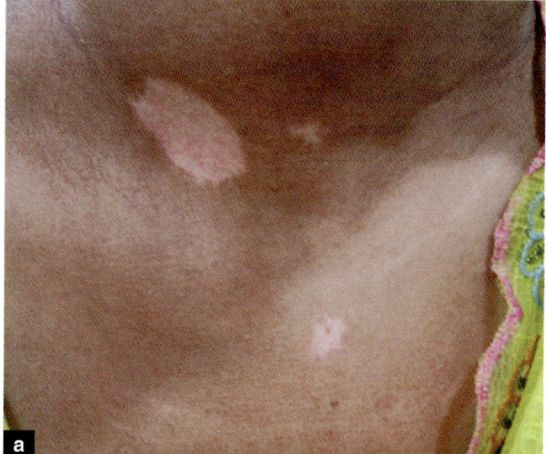

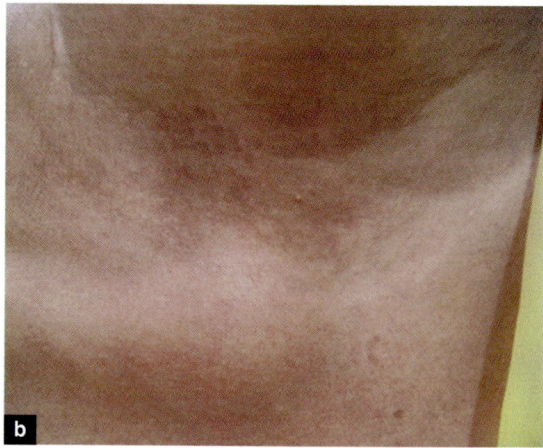

Fig. 2.9a and b: (a) A female patient with vitiligo on the neck. (b) After 3 months of using topical tacrolimus 0.1% with oral PUVA sol (Trimop Forte), complete resolution of the lesion is seen

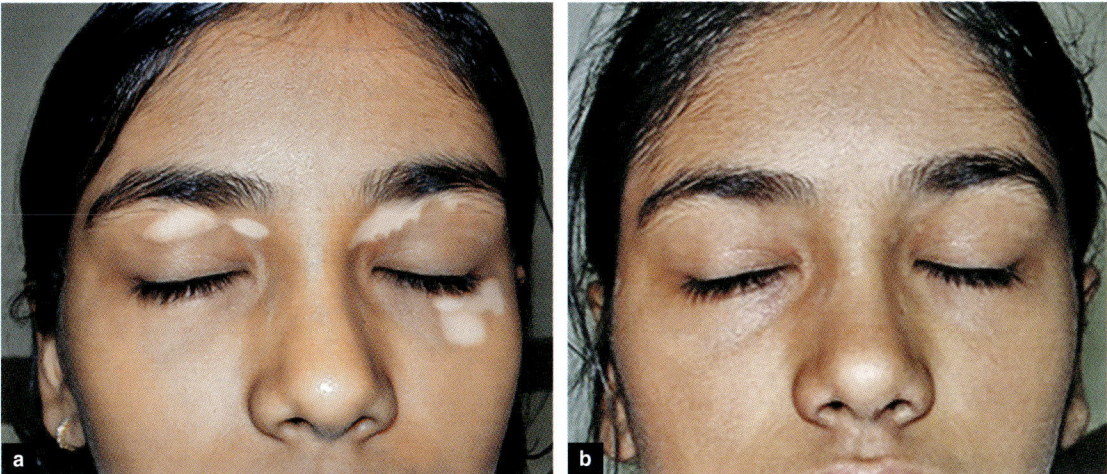

Fig. 2.10a and b: (a) A case of facial vitiligo. (b) After 3 months of tacrolimus 0.1% in the morning and fluticasone propionate 0.05% at night, complete resolution of the lesion is evident

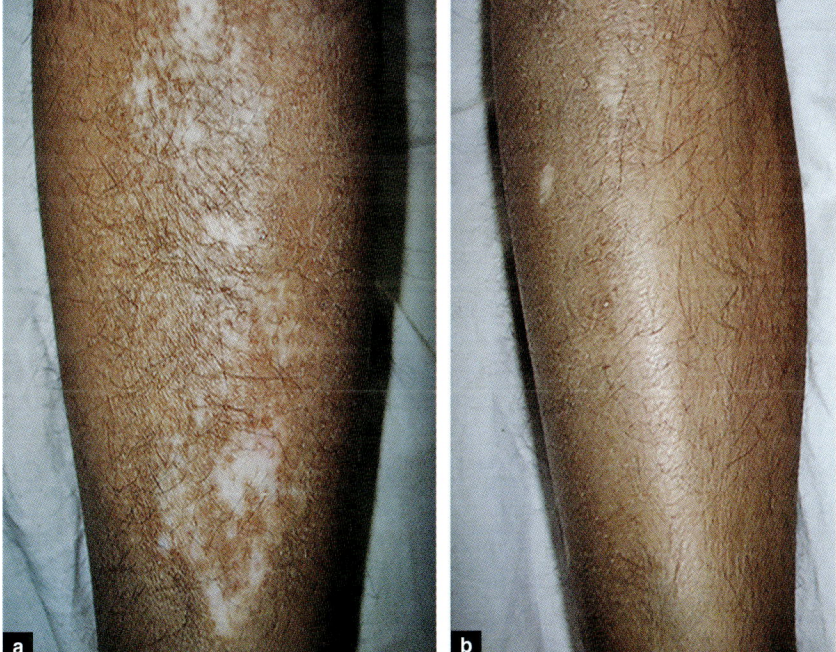

Fig. 2.11a and b: (a) A case of vitiligo on the lower leg. The presence of pigmented hair aids in rapid pigmentation. (b) After 3 months of PUVA with topical Flucort cream at night, near complete pigmentation was seen

option that we follow is to administer Deflazacort (0.25–1 mg/kg) in an alternate day dosage.

2. Topical drugs like tacrolimus 0.1% (Fig. 2.9a and b), topical calcipotriol have been used and are useful if given alternating with topical steroids to avoid side effects. Good results are obtained when these agents are used for facial lesions and/or combined with sun exposure.

3. **Topical psoralen ultraviolet A (PUVA) is** an option but unless supervised tends to cause side effects. Topical 8 methoxyposralen can be administered but requires careful sunlight exposure after 20 minutes beginning with 1 minute alternate day, gradually increasing to 5 minutes over months.

4. **Oral PUVA:** This form of therapy was first used by the Egyptians and Indians. Though in the West, Narrowband-UVB (NB-UVB) therapy is practiced. In India, PUVAsol is still the most cost-effective option (Figs 2.9 and 2.10). Psoralen photo-chemotherapy involves the use of psoralens combined with UVA.

   The psoralen most commonly utilized is 8-methoxypsoralen (8-MOP, methoxsalen), though if sunlight is used 4,5′, 8-trimethylpsoralen (TMP, trioxsalen) should be used. Oral PUVA treatments using 8-MOP (0.4–0.6 mg/kg) are typically administered two times weekly. For patients with vitiligo, the initial dose of UVA is usually 0.5–1.0 J/cm^2, which is gradually increased until minimal asymptomatic erythema of the involved skin occurs.

   A simple protocol, if sunlight is an option, is to give TMP (Neosoralen Forte) 0.6 mg/kg/d and after 2 hours expose to sunlight (11 AM to 3 PM) for 5–10 minutes on an alternate day protocol.

   The response rate of PUVA is variable; although the majority of patients obtain cosmetically acceptable improvement, complete repigmentation is achieved in only a few patients. The total number of PUVA treatments required is generally between 50 and 300.

   A particularly useful treatment regimen is the Pathak regimen, wherein a combination of low-dose 8-methoxy-psoralen 0.3 mg/kg plus trimethylpsoralen 0.6 mg/kg is used followed by sun exposure and helps in achieving a higher rate of repigmentation when compared with the use of either

psoralen alone plus sunlight in various doses.

However, PUVAsol is time-consuming and often ineffective. It should generally not be used for children younger than 9 years. The treatments are 50% to 70% successful in restoring some color on the face, trunk, and upper arms and legs. Again, the hands and feet respond poorly to this method.

The details of phototherapy have been described in Chapter 8.

5. **Other treatment options:** Various other therapies have been tried including topical decapeptide, pseudocatalase, prostaglandins, oral polyvitamins and levamisole but have not been found to be clinically useful as compared to PUVA and topical steroids.

6. Sunscreens can be used to avoid exacerbating the contrast between normal skin and lesions and to protect the lesions, which are sensitive to the sun.

Phototherapy

NB-UVB has become the gold standard of therapy for vitiligo. The mean repigmentation achieved is 41–68% within 3 to 6 months of therapy. It has consistently been shown to be effective, although is not curative.

Surgical/Laser

This is beyond the scope of primary care physicians.

Combination Therapy

Combination therapy may produce higher rates of repigmentation compared to traditional monotherapies. Examples include phototherapy following surgical procedures and topical calcineurin inhibitors (TCIs) or topical corticosteroids used together or with NB-UVB or excimer laser therapy. Although topical vitamin D derivatives are relatively ineffective as monotherapy, these agents may result in additional repigmentation when used in conjunction with phototherapy.

Depigmentation

If attempts at repigmentation do not produce satisfactory results, depigmentation may be attempted in selected patients. Those with extensive vitiligo (more than 50% loss of pigment) may elect to have the remaining skin "bleached" with Benoquin (20% monobenzylether of hydroquinone). The results are permanent.

Traditional Indian Medicines in Vitiligo

One of the myths propagated by the lay media is the role of diet in vitiligo. In fact, lot of clinicians advise against taking vitamin C. One patient of vitiligo complained of recurrent boils and after numerous antibiotic courses did not help, vitamin C was prescribed which helped in reducing his complaint of boils. The patient had not been taking viatmin C in any form for years due to the advice of a clinician, and he still had vitiligo in spite of this dietary intervention.

Another myth is the role of various antioxidants promoted by the pharma industry, which have a small role but may not be relevant in India where the diet is rich in antioxidants.

In light of this, two herbs have been found to have a role in vitiligo. The first is turmeric, which is a powerful antioxidant and can be supplemented in the diet with milk. Numerous studies credit it with its role in preventing oxidative damage and consider it superior to most oral antioxidants. The second is Tulsi (*Ocimum sanctum*) which is a powerful immunomodulatory agent and is useful in conditions like vitiligo. Ample proof on its role is available on pubmed searches (*see* below). We advise against using Ayurvedic medications containing "bhasm" as they invariably contain lead that can cause bone marrow depression.

Flowcharts 2.2 and 2.3 depict the treatment algorithm for segmental and non-segmental vitiligo, respectively. An overview of therapy is given in Table 2.3.

Flowchart 2.2: Treatment algorithm for non-segmental vitiligo

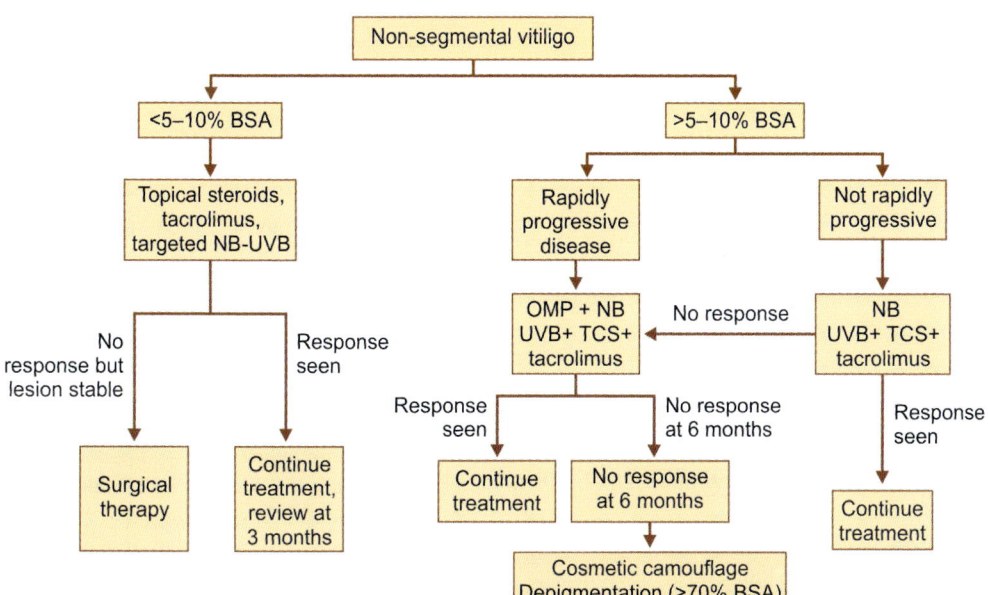

Flowchart 2.3: Treatment algorithm for segmental vitiligo

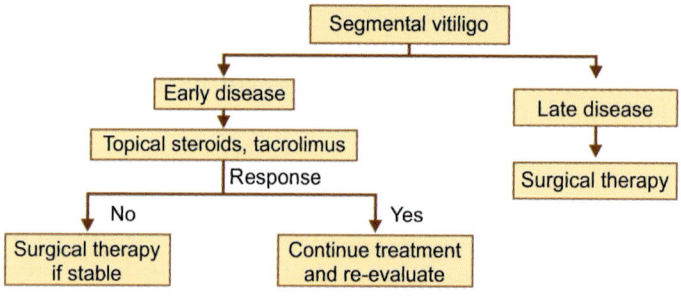

	Medical management	Cosmetic intervention	Laser/surgery
	Table 2.3: Overview of therapy of vitiligo		
Topical	Calcineurin inhibitors Corticosteroids Vitamin D analogs Catalase/superoxide dismutase Topical PUVA[d] MBEH[d] (extensive vitiligo) for complete depigmentation	Camouflage Tattooing	NB-UVB/UVA Excimer laser Grafting
Systemic	PUVA[d] Steroids Immunosuppressants[d]		
Level of care	**Primary**	**Tertiary** Refer to dermatologist	**Tertiary** Refer to dermatologist

[d]Refer to dermatologist

Bibliography

1. Agrawal R, Sandhu SK, Sharma I, Kaur IP. Development and Evaluation of Curcumin-loaded Elastic Vesicles as an Effective Topical Anti-inflammatory Formulation. AAPS Pharm Sci Tech 2014, Oct 16.

2. Alafiatayo AA, Syahida A, Mahmood M. Total anti-oxidant capacity, flavonoid, phenolic acid and polyphenol content in ten selected species of zingiberaceae rhizomes. Afr J Tradit Complement Altern Med 2014 Apr 3;11(3):7–13.

3. Devaraj S, Ismail S, Ramanathan S, Yam MR Investigation of antioxidant and hepatoprotective activity of standardized Curcuma xanthorrhiza rhizome in carbon tetrachloride-induced hepatic damaged rats. Scientific World Jour 2014; 2014: 353128.

4. Evidence-Based, Non-Surgical Treatments for Vitiligo; A Review. Am Jour Clin Dermatol, August 2012, 13 (4), Pp 217–237.

5. Jean-Paul Ortonne and Thierry Passeron. Vitiligo and Other Disorders of Hypopigmentation. 3rd ed. (Bolognia, Dermatology). Elsevier, 2012.

6. Mediratta PK, Sharma KK, Singh S. Evaluation of immunomodulatory potential of ocimum sanctum seed oil and its possible mechanism of action. J Ethnopharmacol 2002 Apr; 80(1):15–20.

7. Mondal S, Varma S, Bamola VD, Naik SN, Mirdha BR, Padhi MM, Mehta N, Mahapatra SC. Double-blinded randomized controlled trial for immunomodulatory effects of Tulsi (Ocimum sanctum Linn.) leaf extract on healthy volunteers. J Ethnopharmacol 2011 Jul 14;136(3):452–6.

8. Pathak MA, Mosher DB, Fitzpatrick TB. Safety and therapeutic effectiveness of 8-methoxypsoralen, 4,5′, 8-trimethylpsoralen and psoralen in vitiligo. Natl Cancer Inst Monogr 1984 Dec; 66: 165–73.

9. Vitiligo. In: Sardana K, Garg VK, Mahajan S, ed. Diagnosis and Management of Skin Diseases: An Evidence Based Approach. Wolters Kluwer, LWW, 2012, 1st edition.

Chemical Depigmentation

It usually occurs as an occupational leucoderma in workers exposed to phenols. p-tertiary-butylphenol is the most important agent amongst these. Other phenols that can cause this condition are monobenzylether of hydroquinone (used in treatment of hyperpigmentation), 4-tertiarybutyl catechol. These cause a lethal effect on melanocytes. The dorsa of hands and feet (Fig. 2.12a and b) are commonly affected though it can occur on sites that are not exposed to the chemical. Treatment of chemical leucoderma is challenging.

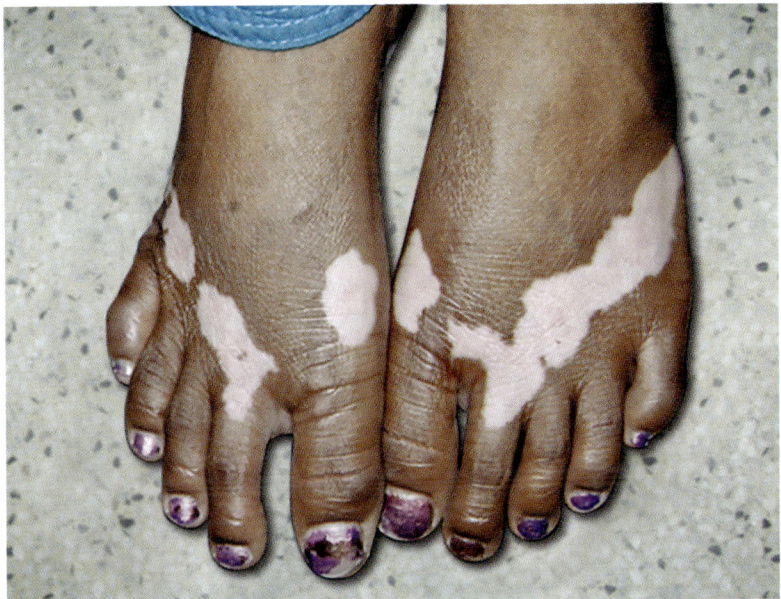

Fig. 2.12a: Chemical leucoderma due to rubber chappals

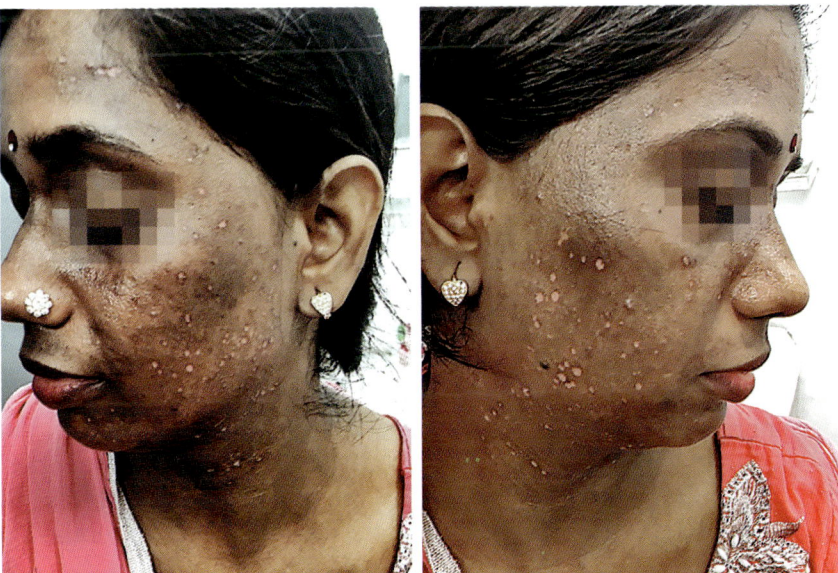

Fig. 2.12b: A patient with hydroquinone-induced depigmentation

INFECTIOUS AND PARASITIC HYPOMELANOSIS

Pityriasis (Tinea) Versicolor

Incidence

Very common in the tropics. Most commonly seen in adolescence and young adulthood.

Lipophilic yeasts, *Malassezia furfur* is a saprophyte. These organisms are normal inhabitants of skin flora but change from the saprophytic form to the hyphae form of *M. furfur*. Depigmentation is due to the fungus producing azelaic acid, which inhibits tyrosinase activity when activated by sunlight.

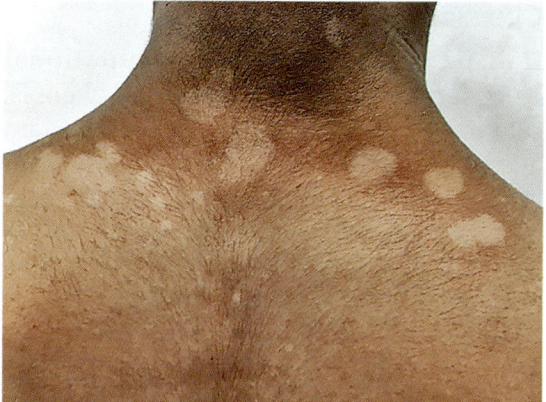

Fig. 2.13: Pityriasis versicolor: Hypopigmented macules over the upper back in a male. On close examination, lesions were found to be scaly.

Risk Factors

Pregnancy, malnutrition, immunosuppression, oral contraception, excess heat and humidity (heavy clothing with perspiration).

Clinical Features

The condition is common in early twenties and rare in childhood. Pityriasis versicolor is characterized by discrete or confluent, scaly, discolored or depigmented areas, mainly on the upper trunk, neck, face, arms and thighs (Figs 2.13 to 2.15). Trunk is the most common site; other sites include face, upper arm and groin. Facial lesions are more common in children. In the untanned white skin, the affected areas are darker than normal. In the sun-tanned subject, the abnormal skin is commonly paler, as it usually is in black people. Lesions may sometimes show some degree of atrophy.

Differential Diagnosis

Vitiligo, secondary syphilis, pityriasis alba, seborrheic dermatitis and pityriasis rosea.

Investigations

Diagnosis is primarily clinical and is confirmed by demonstrating the hyphae and spores of *Malassezia furfur* using 10%

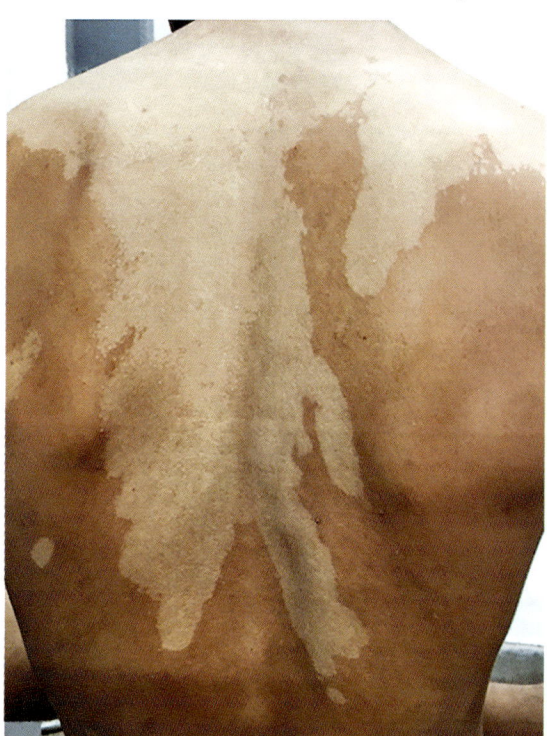

Fig. 2.14: Extensive pityriasis versicolor over the back in a young male

potassium hydroxide. Large, blunt hyphae and thick-walled, budding spores forming a 'spaghetti and meatballs' appearance should be observed under the low-powered lens of a microscope.

Histology is depicted in Fig. 2.15b.

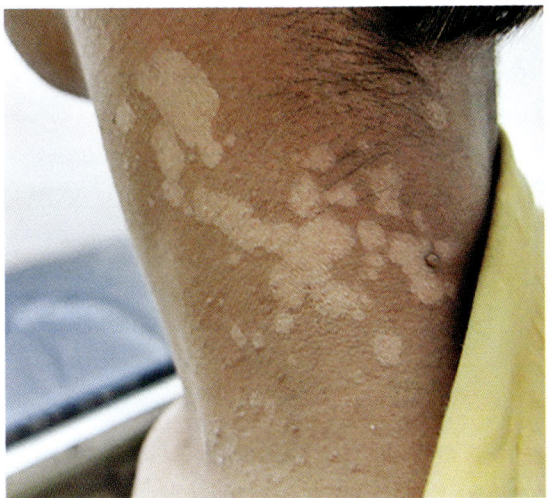

Fig. 2.15a: Scaly macules on the neck in a case of pityriasis versicolor

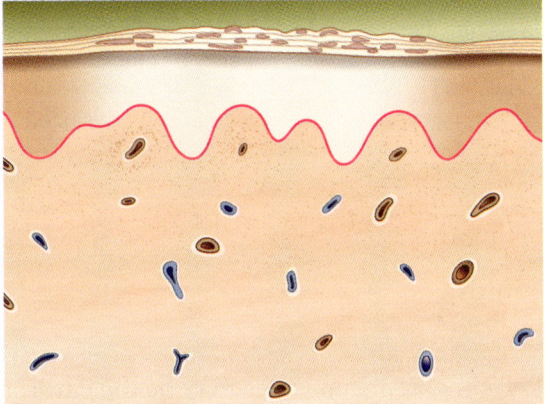

Fig. 2.15b: Tinea versicolor. Epidermis—mild hyperkeratosis; hyphae and spores, decreased pigmentation. Dermis—normal

Treatment

Non-pharmacological therapy: Sunlight accelerates repigmentation of hypopigmented areas.

Patient counselling/advise:
- Patients (or caregivers) should be advised that it is a treatable fungal infection with benign lesions and that treatment may need to be continued for up to 4 weeks.
- Optimal compliance is necessary to improve eradication rates.

- Skin may not regain its natural pigment for several months after successful eradication of the fungus.
- Recurrence will occur in over 80% of previously cured cases over 2 years. It is important for patients to understand that recurrence does not mean lack of efficacy of treatment; otherwise they may become frustrated.

Topical agents:
- Topical imidazole antifungals (e.g. clotrimazole, econazole, miconazole) form the mainstay of treatment and should be first-line therapy for up to 4 weeks.
- Selenium sulfide 2.5% suspension applied from neck to waist and other affected area(s), rinsed thoroughly with water after 15 minutes; applied once daily for 7 days; and repeated weekly for 1 month, then monthly for maintenance.

Systemic agents: Oral treatment should only be used in recalcitrant cases in patients who have not responded to topical therapy. Effective agents are ketoconazole 200 mg OD for 7 days, or single 400 mg dose (cure rate >80%), fluconazole 400 mg given as a single dose (cure rate >70% at 3 weeks after treatment) or itraconazole 200 mg/day for 7 days.

Chemoprophylaxis: Systemic prophylaxis is reserved for highly recurrent cases that are severe enough to cause significant distress and is not routinely recommended. Itraconazole (200 mg orally, twice daily, 1 day per month) or ketoconazole (400 mg orally, every 14 days or 200 mg orally, for 3 consecutive days per month) is advised.

Course and Complications

The prognosis is good, with death of the fungus usually occurring within 3 to 4 weeks

Table 2.4: Overview of treatment of pityriasis versicolor

	Medical management	Cosmetic intervention	Laser/surgery
Topical	Topical imidazole antifungals (e.g. clotrimazole, econazole, miconazole) BD application up to 4 weeks	None	None
Systemic	Ketoconazole: 200 mg orally, daily for 7 days, or 400 mg as a single dose Itraconazole: 200 mg orally, daily for 7 days, or 400 mg as a single dose Fluconazole: 400 mg orally, as a single dose, or 150 mg/week for 4 weeks		
Level of care	**Primary** Good nutrition (eating 6–8 servings of fruits and vegetables a day, with limited intake of sugar and simple carbohydrates) Good hygiene (controlling excessive perspiration) Cool climate (reducing heat and humidity in the living environment)	**Tertiary** If recurrence occurs and treatment compliance is optimal, then referral to a dermatologist is indicated	**Tertiary** Refer to dermatologist. If deterioration occurs, referral is indicated because comorbidity needs to be excluded

of treatment; however, recurrence is common.

Table 2.4 gives details about the therapy.

Bibliography

1. Hay RJ, Ashbee HR. Mycology. In: Burns T, Breathnach S, Cox N, Griffiths C, edn. Rook's Textbook of Dermatology. 8th edn. Oxford: Blackwell Science; 2010. Chapter 36, p. 36.10–36.12.
2. Janik MP, Heffernan MR. Yeast infections: Candidiasis and tinea (pityriasis) versicolor. In: Wolff K, Goldsmith LA, Katz SI, Gilchrest BA, Paller AS, Leffell DJ et. al. eds. Fitzpatrick's Dermatology in General Medicine. 7th edn., Chapter 189, p. 1828–30.
3. Kailini JR, Riaz F, Khachemoune A. Tinea versicolor in dark-skinned individuals. Int J Dermatol 2014 Feb;53(2):137–41.
4. Pedrosa AF, Lisboa C, Gongalves Rodrigues A. Malassezia infections: A medical conundrum. J Am Acad Dermatol 2014 Jul;71(1):170–6.

Leprosy

Clinical Features

Hypomelanotic macules may be the earliest expression of lepromatous leprosy. The lesions are usually small, multiple, subtle and ill-defined; they may be difficult to recognize, particularly in lightly pigmented skin. The face, extremities and buttocks are favored, and the warmer parts of the body are usually spared. There is little or no anhidrosis or loss of sensation. Later, nodules or diffuse infiltration of the skin appear.

There are various types of leprosy but broadly two types have been described—tuberculoid and lepromatous types. The hypopigmented patches of tuberculoid leprosy are much different from those of lepromatous leprosy.

Tuberculoid lesions have discrete edges and can be quite large, up to 30 cm in diameter. Initial lesions may have minimal infiltration with hypopigmentation (Fig. 2.16a). A raised border, uniform infiltration or a characteristic pebbled appearance may be observed. The surface can be slightly scaly, dry or minimally atrophic. The lesions are asymmetrically distributed on the posterolateral aspects of the extremities, back, buttocks and face. There is associated loss of hair, anhidrosis, and loss of tactile and heat sensations.

In **borderline** (dimorphous) leprosy, plaques and annular lesions are more common than hypomelanotic macules (Fig. 2.16b); the latter, if present, have ill-defined borders and are faintly visible. A "Swiss cheese" appearance with erythematous annular lesions and hypomelanotic areas, all bound by vague outer borders, characterizes this form of leprosy.

In **indeterminate** leprosy, the macules are usually hypomelanotic, but they may also be erythematous; hypoesthesia may be present. They are asymmetrically distributed and favor exposed sites.

Diagnosis

A case of leprosy is diagnosed by eliciting cardinal signs of leprosy through systematic clinical (and wherever required bacteriological) examination.

- At least one of the following cardinal (unique and very important) signs must be present to diagnose leprosy.
  a. Hypopigmented or reddish skin lesion(s) with definite sensory deficit.
  b. Involvement of the peripheral nerves, as demonstrated by definite thickening with loss of sensation and weakness of the corresponding muscles of the hands, feet or eyes.
  c. Demonstration of *M. leprae* in the lesions.

  The first two cardinal signs can be identified by clinical examination alone while the third can be identified by examination of a slit skin smear.
- A person with cardinal signs of leprosy and yet to complete full course of multidrug therapy (MDT) may be called "case of leprosy" (Table 2.5).

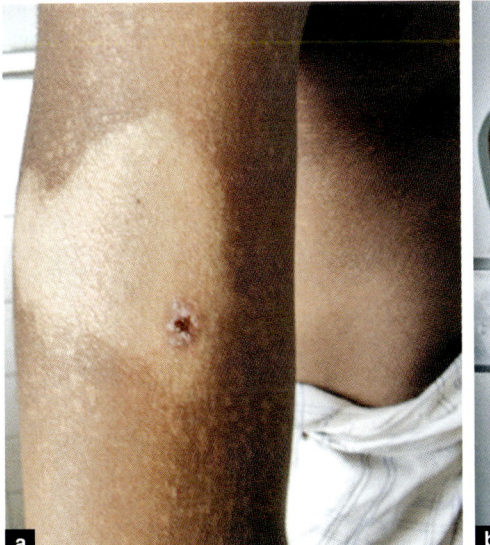
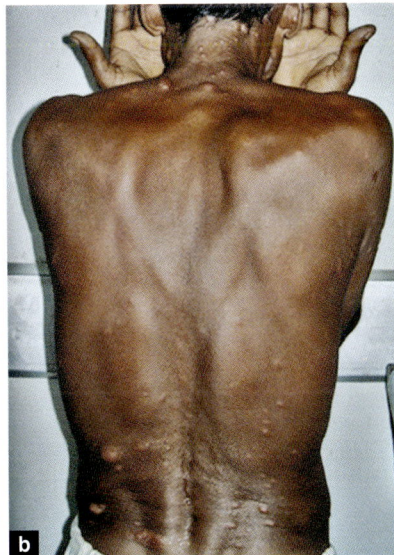

Fig. 2.16a and b: (a) TT leprosy with a large hypopigmented macule; (b) BL leprosy: Papules, nodules, and faint hypopigmented macules

Table 2.5: Criteria for grouping

Characteristic	PB (pauci bacillary)	MB (multi-bacillary)
1. Skin lesions	1–5 lesions	6 and above
2. Peripheral nerve	No nerve/only one nerve involvement	More than one nerve
3. Skin smear	Negative at all sites	Positive at any site

Treatment

Treatment usually, but not always, results in repigmentation of the hypomelanotic macules. In India, the regimen depends largely on the type of leprosy as given below.

The treatment of leprosy is in the form of multi-drug therapy (Table 2.6) which is the combination of two or three of the following drugs:

a. Cap. Rifampicin
b. Tab. Dapsone
c. Cap. Clofazimine
i. MDT kills the bacilli (*M. leprae*) in the body and thus stops the progression of the disease and prevents further complications.
ii. As the *M. leprae* are killed, the patient becomes non-infectious and thus the spread of infection in the body is

Table 2.6: MDT drugs used in leprosy

	Drugs and (adult)	Dosage	Frequency of administration	Criteria for RFT		
MB leprosy	Rifampicin Dapsone Clofazimine Clofazimine	600 mg 100 mg 300 mg 50 mg	Once monthly Daily Once monthly Daily	Completion of 12 monthly pulses		
PB leprosy	Rifampicin Dapsone	600 mg 100 mg	Once montly Daily	Completion of 6 monthly pulses		
MDT regimen (Child: 10–14 years of age)						
MB leprosy	Rifampicin Dapsone Clofazimine Clofazimine	450 mg 50 mg 150 mg 50 mg	Once monthly Daily Once monthly Every other day	Completion of 12 monthly pulses		
PB leprosy	Rifampicin Dapsone	450 mg 50 mg	Once monthly Daily	Completion of 6 monthly pulses		

reduced. Moreover, spread of infection to other persons is also reduced.

iii. Using a combination of two or three drugs instead of one drug alone will ensure effective cure and there are no chances of development of resistance to the drugs.

Based on the grouping, the patients can be given any one of the standard MDT regimens mentioned below. In children, the dose may be adjusted suitably.

When the patient has completed the required number of doses (monthly pulses) of standard MDT regimens, s/he is released from treatment—RFT.

The duration depends on the spectrum for PB × 6 months MB × 12 months.

MDT regimen (children): The appropriate dose for children under 10 years of age can be decided on the basis of body weight.

Bibliography

Training Manual for Medical Officer Central Leprosy Division, Directorate General of Health Services, Nirman Bhawan, New Delhi National.

POST-KALA-AZAR DERMAL LEISHMANIASIS (PKDL)

Small hypomelanotic macules in a symmetric distribution that favors the upper trunk, face and arms constitute the prenodular stage of the disease (Fig. 2.17a). They can be associated in classic cases with nodules (Fig. 2.17b and c).

As leprosy and PKDL may overlap in the clinical manifestations, a protocol for differentiation is shown in Flowchart 2.4.

The lesions become elevated over a period of months to years. Total repigmentation following systemic treatment with antimonials is almost impossible to achieve.

Idiopathic Guttate Hypomelanosis

Clinical Features

Idiopathic guttate hypomelanosis (IGH—white spots on the arms and legs) is characterized by 2 to 5 mm porcelain white spots with sharply demarcated borders. They are located on the exposed areas of hands, forearms, and lower legs of middle-aged and older people (Fig. 2.18a and b).

Patients have signs of early ageing and sun exposure, including seborrheic keratoses, lentigines, and xerosis in the same areas. A subset of these patients has lesions unrelated to sun exposure. The condition is asymptomatic.

The pathogenesis of IGH is not clearly known. It could be a part of the normal ageing process. Chronic exposure to UV radiation can be another factor as lesions occur on sun-exposed sites. Diagnosis is mainly clinical. Wood's lamp examination can be used to confirm the diagnosis.

Dermoscopy can be used to differentiate it from vitiligo (Fig. 2.18c).

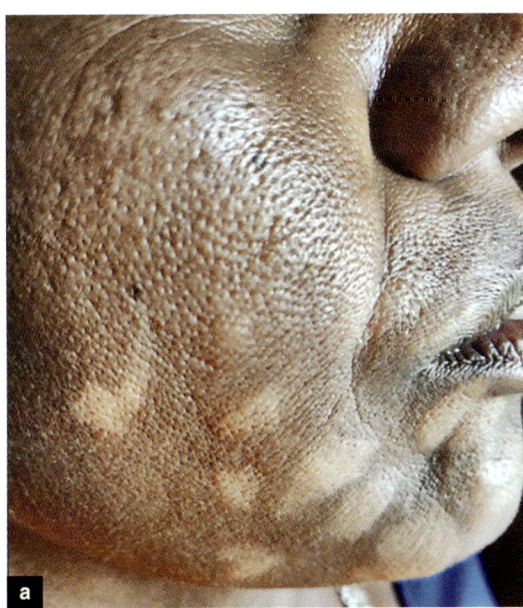

Fig. 2.17a: Hypopigmented macules—PKDL (Dr Gaurish Laad, Goa)

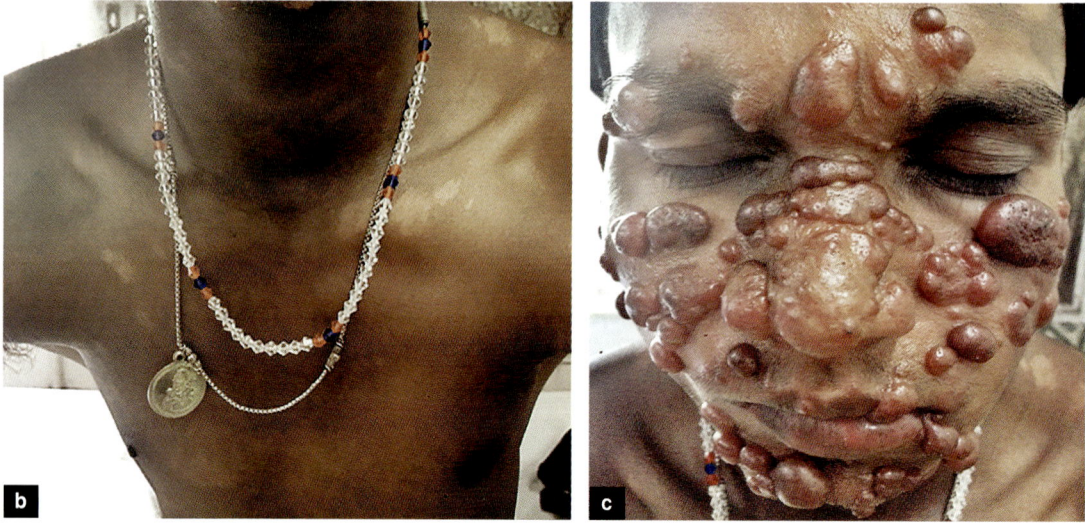

Fig. 2.17b and c: (b) Multiple hypomelanotic macules over the upper trunk in a patient with post-kala-azar dermal leishmaniasis. Lesions generally do not respond to treatment. (c) Multiple erythematous translucent nodules in the same patient

Flowchart 2.4: Common flowchart for leprosy and kala-azar workers

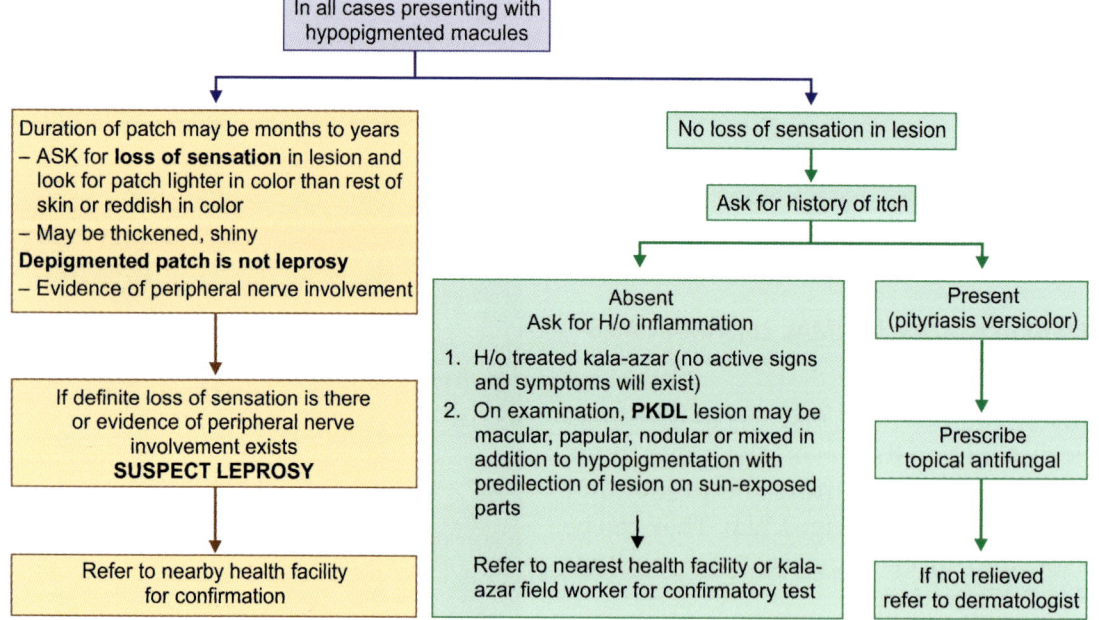

Treatment

Treatment with tretinoin for 4 months restores the elasticity, with a partial restoration of pigmentation. Cryotherapy for 3 to 5 seconds is also effective. Topical steroids and tacrolimus can also be used.

Progressive Macular Hypomelanosis

Progressive macular hypomelanosis (PMH) is a common acquired hypopigmented disorder that is often misdiagnosed. It is characterized by ill-defined round hypopigmented macules affecting the trunk in young

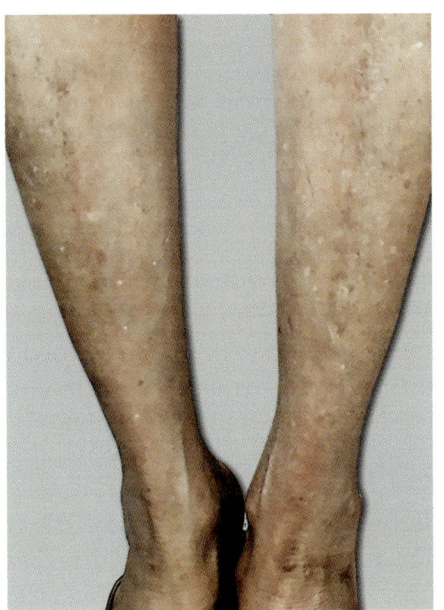

Fig. 2.18a: Idiopathic guttate hypomelanosis: Sharply demarcated depigmented macules

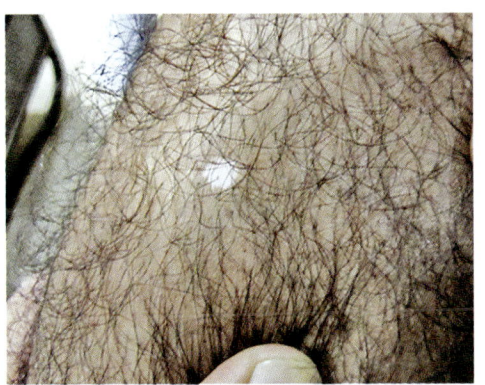

Fig. 2.18b: Idiopathic guttate hypomelanosis (IGH)

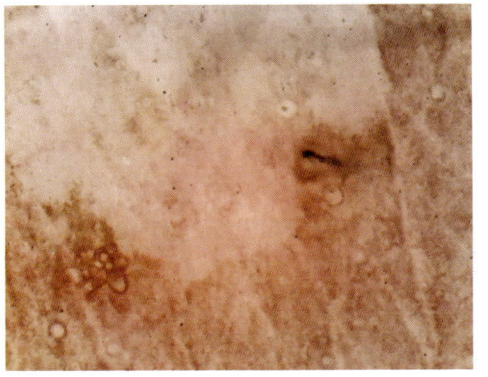

Fig. 2.18c: IGH in patient with vitiligo showing a petaloid pattern on dermoscopy

adults. The condition may progress over time or remain stable but rarely regresses.

Propionibacterium species has been postulated as a causative agent. Clindamycin and benzoyl peroxide have been found to be beneficial. Phototherapy has also been tried with good improvement.

Nutritional Hypomelanosis

In kwashiorkor, which is due to severe protein deficiency, the skin initially becomes erythematous to red-brown in color with marked desquamation. Both hypomelanosis and patchy post-inflammatory hypermelanosis can be seen, with striking pigmentary changes in florid cases. The hypomelanosis usually begins on the face. The hair is dry and lusterless, and it may become light red-brown in color. Upon resumption of dietary protein intake, the skin repigments slowly. Diffuse pigmentary dilution due to deficiencies of copper or selenium have also been reported.

Bibliography

Pigmentation Disorders. In: Sardana K, Garg VK, Mahajan S, ed. Diagnosis and Management of Skin Diseases: An Evidence Based Approach, Wolters Kluwer, LWW 1st edn., 2012.

3. RARE DISORDERS

ALBINISM

Clinical Features

Oculocutaneous albinism (OCA) consists of a group of genetic disorders characterized by diffuse pigmentary dilution due to a partial or total absence of melanin pigment within melanocytes of the skin, hair follicles, and eyes. The number of epidermal and follicular melanocytes is normal. Hypopigmentation involving primarily the retinal pigment epithelium is termed ocular albinism (OA).

It is of six types depending on the gene involved. OCA type 1 is the commonest and is due to mutation in tyrosinase gene TYR. The severity of clinical features vary according to the type of albinism. Pigmentation of skin, hair, and eyes is reduced. There are associated ophthalmological anomalies like nystagmus, hypopigmented iris, reduced visual acuity and refractive errors. The retinal pigment epithelium shows reduced pigmentation. Photophobia is marked. Intelligence and development are normal.

There is predisposition to skin cancers due to increased sensitivity to UV radiation.

Treatment

No specific treatment is available. Photoprotection (sunscreens, hats, clothing, sun avoidance) is mandatory in patients who have minimal or no pigmentation, in order to avoid cutaneous photocarcinogenesis, in particular the development of squamous cell carcinomas.

Bibliography

Pigmentation Disorders. In: Sardana K, Garg VK, Mahajan S, ed. Diagnosis and Management of Skin Diseases: An Evidence Based Approach, Welters Kluwer, LWW 2012, 1st edn.

PIEBALDISM

Piebaldism is an uncommon autosomal dominant disorder characterized by poliosis and congenital, stable, circumscribed areas of leukoderma due to an absence of melanocytes within involved sites.

Clinical Features

The leukoderma has a characteristic distribution pattern that favors the central anterior trunk, mid-extremities, central forehead, and mid-frontal portion of the scalp; the latter results in a white forelock (Fig. 2.19). The lesions are present at birth and classically spare the posterior midline. The white forelock, which is present in 80–90% of patients, is the most familiar feature

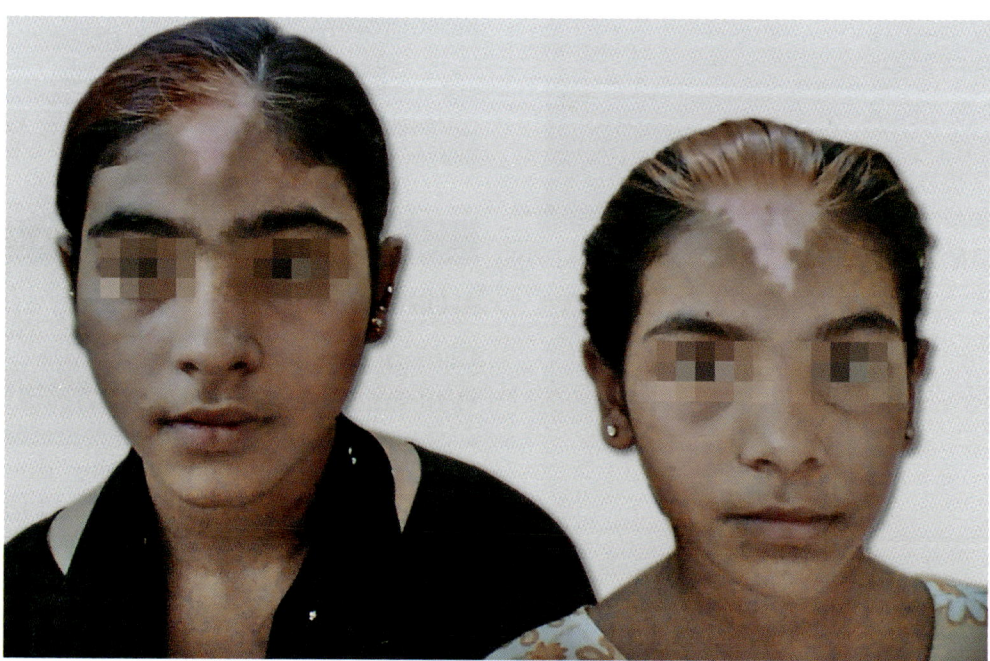

Fig. 2.19: White forelock and characteristic triangular amelanotic patch on the mid-forehead in a case of Piebaldism

of piebaldism. However, its absence does not exclude the diagnosis. All the hairs of the forelock are white, and the underlying skin is also amelanotic.

This depigmented patch is midline in location, triangular or diamond-shaped, and often symmetrical. The apex can reach the vertex posteriorly and the affected area may extend to the root of the nose and includes the medial third of the eyebrows; involvement of the nose is rare. Normally, pigmented and hyperpigmented macules and patches (ranging from a few millimeters to several centimeters in diameter) are typically apparent within the leukodermic patches (Fig. 2.19).

Differential Diagnosis

Piebaldism should be differentiated from vitiligo. In the former, depigmented patches are present since birth and remain stable throughout life. The lesions have a characteristic medial distribution. In patients with associated sensorineural deafness and dysmorphic features, diagnosis of Waardenburg syndrome should be considered.

Treatment

Autografts of normal skin into amelanotic areas, including grafting of autologous melanocytes are a therapeutic option but this typically requires multiple procedures. Cosmetic products can be used to camouflage affected areas and protection against sunburn is also necessary.

Bibliography

Pigmentation Disorders. In: Sardana K, Garg VK, Mahajan S, edn. Diagnosis and Management of Skin Diseases: An Evidence based Approach, Wolters Kluwer, LWW, 1st edn., 2012.

TUBEROUS SCLEROSIS COMPLEX

The tuberous sclerosis complex (TSC) represents an autosomal dominant disorder characterized by hamartomas in multiple organs, most commonly the skin, brain, eye, heart, and kidney.

Clinical Features

The classic TSC triad of facial angiofibromas (adenoma sebaceum), seizures, and mental deficits is preceded by the appearance of white macules.

Hypomelanotic macules are often evident at birth or during the neonatal period and as most infants are fair-skinned at birth are often missed. The great majority of patients have 2–20 hypomelanotic macules, with 50% having fewer than six and 50% having six or more macules. Lesions may be polygonal, lance-ovate, "thumbprint-like", guttate (confetti-like) or rarely segmental (Fig. 2.20). The macules and patches are a dull white color (hypomelanotic), not the "pure-white" color (amelanotic) of vitiligo.

Diagnosis

If an infant has three or more hypopigmented macules, a diagnosis of TSC should be considered and (if there is no history of seizures) echocardiography performed as an initial investigation. The presence of three

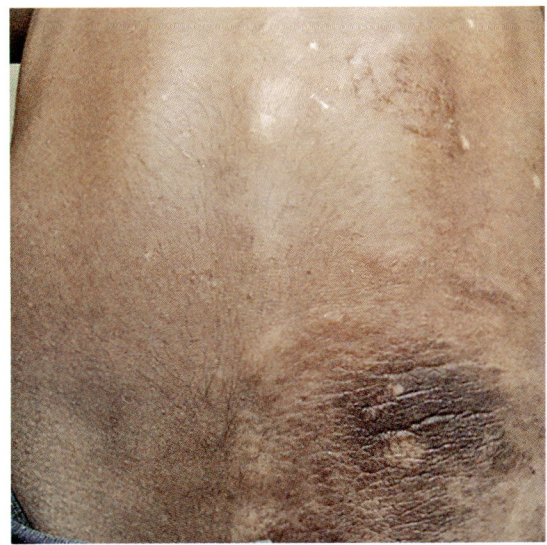

Fig. 2.20: A case of tuberous sclerosis with hypomelanotic macules and a raised shagreen patch

or more hypomelanotic macules, especially if lance-ovate in shape, raises the possibility of TSC. The combination of white macules and seizures increases the likelihood of TSC.

1. Although the presence of only one or two hypopigmented macules or patches in an otherwise healthy infant does not completely exclude TSC, the diagnosis of nevus depigmentosus is much more likely.
2. It is usually fairly easy to distinguish vitiligo, given its characteristic distribution pattern and the pure-white color.
3. Post-inflammatory hypopigmentation is typically easily excluded by the lack of preceding or concurrent inflammatory or trauma-induced lesions.
4. Nevus anemicus is readily distinguished by its "disappearance" upon diascopy; in addition, vigorous rubbing or application of ice produces erythema in the hypopigmented lesions of TSC but not in nevus anemicus.
5. Hypomelanotic macules may be observed in patients with ataxia telangiectasia (likely reflecting "pigmentary mosaicism").

Treatment

There is no treatment but such cases should be referred to dermatologists.

Bibliography

Pigmentation Disorders. In: Sardana K, Garg VK, Mahajan S, eds. Diagnosis and Management of Skin Diseases: An Evidence Based Approach, Wolters Kluwer, LWW, 1st edn., 2012.

HYPOMELANOSIS OF ITO (HOI)

Clinical Features

Newborns with hypomelanosis of Ito have bizarre hypopigmented swirls on their skin that follow Blaschko's lines (Fig. 2.21). These are imaginary lines that are predictive of embryonic fusion lines.

The hypopigmentation may be quite extensive, involving an entire half of the body, or in some circumstances it may even be found bilaterally. Patients with hypomelanosis of Ito may have associated neurologic, skeletal, and/or ocular abnormalities. Because it is not a single entity but a cutaneous sign of mosaicism, the exact incidence is unknown.

Diagnosis

The differential diagnosis of hypomelanosis of Ito is the same as that for hypopigmented macules, but it is distinguished by the whorled pattern following Blaschko's lines and by involvement of an extensive portion of the body.

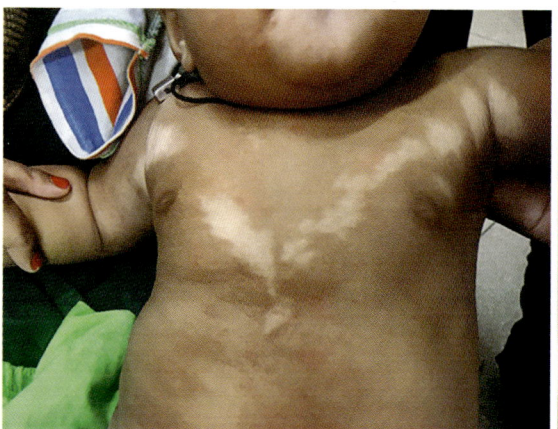 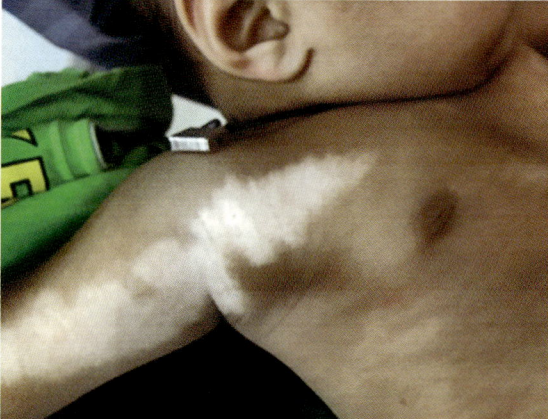

Fig. 2.21a: Hypomelanosis of Ito: "S" shaped whorled pattern of hypopigmented macules along lines of Blaschko in an infant

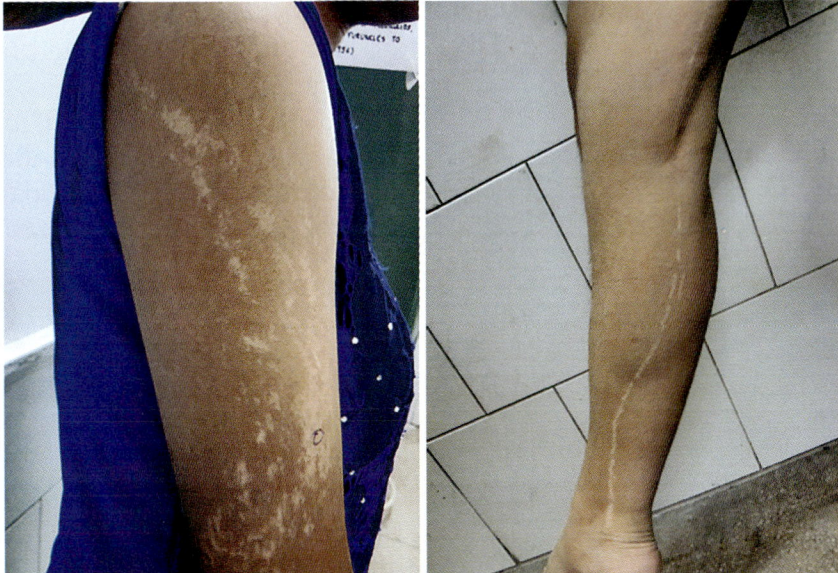

Fig. 2.21b: Hypomelanosis of Ito: Hypopigmented macules along lines of Blaschko present since birth in a girl

As some cases may not be HOI, but segmental nevus depigmentosus, such cases may be referred, as the systemic associations of HOI may be alarming.

Treatment

As with the other hypopigmented and depigmented problems, no treatment is available for the pigmentary changes. Associated neurologic, skeletal, or ophthalmologic problems should be referred to the appropriate specialist.

The clinician should inform the parents that the number of infants who will have associated problems is unknown. They should also be told that no specific genetic defect has been identified.

Bibliography

Pigmentation Disorders. In: Sardana K, Garg VK, Mahajan S, eds. Diagnosis and Management of Skin Diseases: An Evidence Based Approach, Wolters Kluwer, LWW, 1st edn., 2012.

NEVUS DEPIGMENTOSUS

The name is a bit of a misnomer, as the areas of leukoderma are actually hypomelanotic rather than amelanotic. This is the most important differentiating feature from vitiligo. In fact, many cases are misdiagnosed as vitiligo and this causes a lot of mental stress to the patients and their parents.

Clinical Features

Nevus depigmentosus generally presents at birth, or within several months after birth as a unilateral, localized, quasidermatomal patch of hypopigmentation (Fig. 2.22).

The lesions classically appear as breaking apart into smaller macules at the periphery (Fig. 2.23). A block-like variant of nevus depigmentosus, also referred to as the hypopigmented form of the "segmental pigmentation disorder", typically features midline demarcation and less distinct lateral borders.

Treatment

As with the other forms of congenital hypopigmentation, there is no effective treatment. Because of the hypopigmentation in these areas, they should be protected from excess UVR. Parents should be informed of

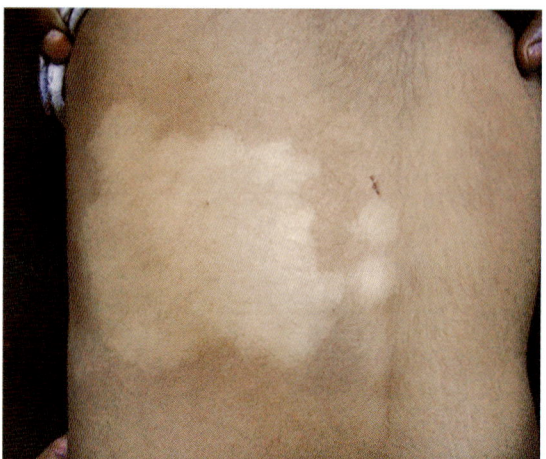

Fig. 2.22: Nevus depigmentosus. Hypomelanotic patch with a decrease but not absence of pigmentation. The segmental nature can be confused with hypomelanosis of Ito

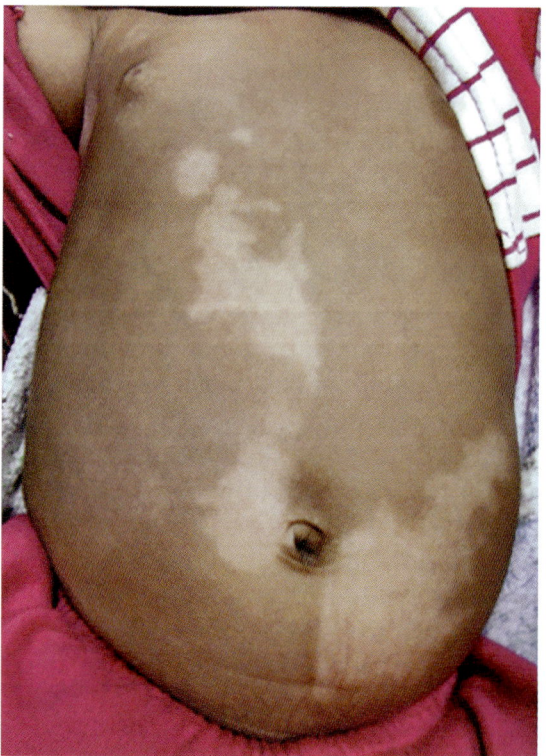

Fig. 2.23: A hypopigmented stable macule on the trunk (nevus depigmentosus)

the chronicity and benign nature of this birthmark. They should be told that the involved area of skin will be more sensitive

to UVR than the child's normal skin and that the area should be protected from excess sunlight.

As the lesion is permanent, it is useful to tell patients to use it as an identification mark in documents, which helps to allay any fears they may have of its spread!

Bibliography

Pigmentation Disorders. In: Sardana K, Garg VK, Mahajan S, eds. Diagnosis and Management of Skin Diseases: An Evidence Based Approach, Wolters Kluwer, LWW, 1st edn., 2012.

NEVUS ANEMICUS

The condition presents at birth or early in childhood. It persists into adulthood and remains unchanged.

Clinical Features

This condition is seen most often on the trunk. The lesion is characterized by a single patch of pale skin with irregular borders. The border can be obliterated by blanching the surrounding skin.

Treatment

No treatment is effective.

Bibliography

Pigmentation Disorders. In: Sardana K, Garg VK, Mahajan S, eds. Diagnosis and Management of Skin Diseases: An Evidence Based Approach, Wolters Kluwer, LWW, 1st edn., 2012.

HALO NEVUS/SUTTON NEVUS

It is characterized by a halo of hypo-pigmentation that develops around a central pigmented nevi (Fig. 2.24a and b). It is usually seen over the trunk in young people and is more common in patients with vitiligo. Pathogenesis of vitiligo and halo nevus is completely distinct. It can also occur around a lesion of malignant melanoma.

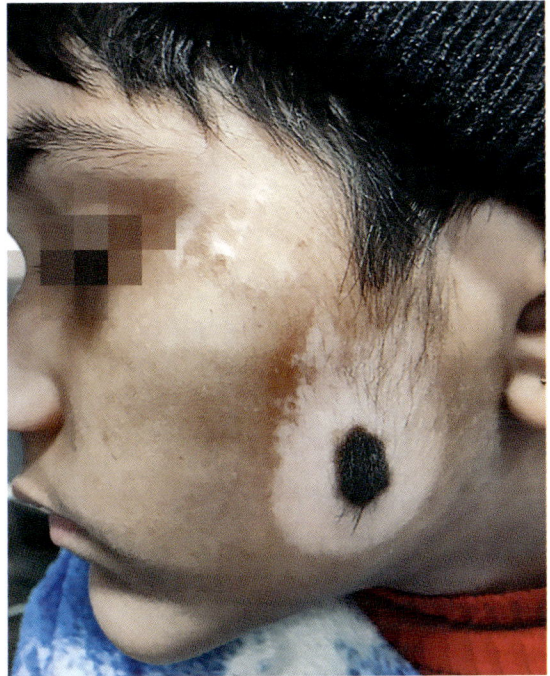

Fig. 2.24a: Sutton nevus/halo nevus: A child with vitiligo with halo of depigmentation around melanocytic naevus

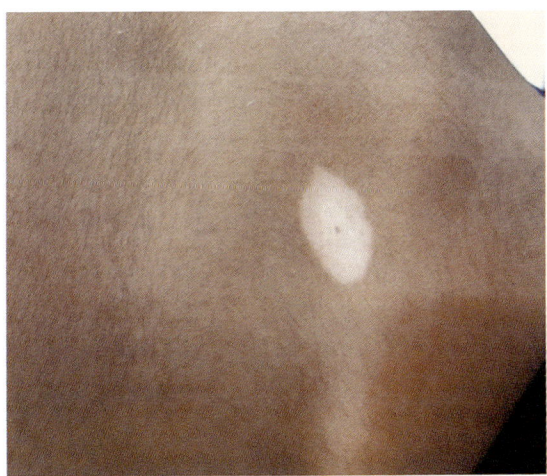

Fig. 2.24b: A case of halo nevus where the central nevus has nearly disappeared leaving a depigmented macule

The lesions may remain stable or repigment spontaneously. Although the pathogenesis is still unknown, the destruction of melanocytes could be due to an immune response that is cell mediated.

Melanoma-associated leukoderma: Hypopigmented or depigmented macules develop at sites distant to the site of the primary melanoma. The condition can be differentiated from vitiligo as the lesions are asymmetric and start on the trunk and spread later to the face and extremities. But in vitiligo, lesions are symmetrical and start from the face and extremities. The diagnosis is mainly clinical though Wood's lamp can be used as an aide in diagnosis.

It occurs due to cell-mediated immune reaction against common antigens on normal and malignant melanocytes.

MORPHEA

This is a chronic autoimmune disease characterized by sclerosis of skin. Morphea arises from genetic background that increases disease susceptibility along with other etiological factors such as infections, drugs, etc.

Clinical Features

Circumscribed/localized lesions, limited to epidermis, dermis, subcutis, fascia, and muscle.

Linear morphea, pansclerotic and mixed variant.

This begins as an erythematous plaque, hypopigmentation develops at the center of lesion, surrounded by an erythematous or violaceous border (inflammatory stage). Sclerosis develop centrally (Fig. 2.25) and this leads to a shiny white color as the lesion expands with surrounding hyperpigmentation (sclerotic stage). In the atrophic stage, cigarette paper wrinkling can be present.

Investigations

- Autoantibodies are reported in cases of morphea—antinuclear antibody (30–80%), dsDNA, antihistone, etc.
- MRI can assess the depth of involvement.

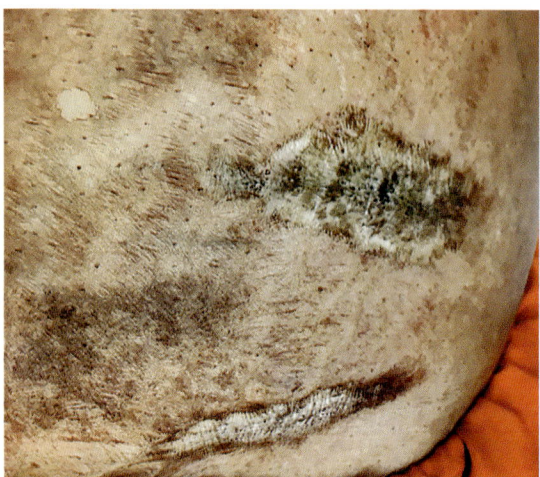

Fig. 2.25: Sclerotic bound down plaques of morphea on the trunk

- Ultrasound can monitor tissue thickness, loss of subcutaneous fat and muscle.
- Histopathology depends on two factors—stage and area sampled. At the inflammatory border, vascular changes are present, e.g. vessel wall thickening. In later stages, inflammatory infiltrate reduces, epidermis is normal, rete ridges are reduced, edema is absent and capillaries are reduced (Breathnach 2010).

Diagnosis

Confirmation requires a biopsy. However, to assess the depth of involvement, MRI should be done.

Treatment

For superficial and localized forms, topical treatments, such as tacrolimus and high-potency corticosteroids, topical calcipotriene or phototherapy with narrow-band UVB, UVB, UVA or UVA-1 are advised.

- Active lesions are treated with superpotent topical or intralesional corticosteroids which may help to reduce inflammation and prevent progression.
- Tacrolimus 0.1% ointment may be a useful first-line agent for active, limited plaque morphea.

- Topical calcipotriene with nightly occlusion (e.g. with plastic wrap) increases penetration of the medication. The combination of topical calcipotriol with betamethasone dipropionate has also been reported to be effective.

Generalized or Deep Morphea

- Systemic corticosteroids are useful in the inflammatory phases of morphea but are not of use in established sclerosis.
- Other drugs, which have been used for generalized morphea, include mycophenolate mofetil, cyclosporine, hydroxychloroquine and methotrexate.
- Phototherapy may be beneficial as a second-line therapy for refractory or severe disease, or as a first-line therapy for patients with generalized morphea given its low side effect profile compared to immunosuppressive agents. As UVA1 wavelengths penetrate deeper into the dermis, this modality is particularly effective in the treatment of morphea. Combination regimens of UV therapy with topical corticosteroids or calcipotriene may be more effective than either therapy alone.
- Other approaches are aimed at altering the cytokine milieu. These include topical halofuginone (transforming growth factor-beta synthesis inhibitor), TNF-α inhibitors, imatinib, and thalidomide (interleukin 12 and tumor necrosis factor-alpha inducer).

An overview of the treatment modalities is given in Table 2.7.

POST-INFECTIOUS HYPOMELANOSIS

1. Treponematoses

Pinta

Hypomelanotic lesions occur during the late phase of the disease, a few months to several years after the appearance of secondary lesions.

	Medical management	Cosmetic intervention	Laser/surgery
Table 2.7: Overview of treatment modalities of morphea			
Topical	Ultra-potent topical corticosteroids Intralesional triamcinolone Pimecrolimus Tacrolimus Calcipotriol		Surgical correction
Systemic	Immunosuppressive agents[d] Oral corticosteroids Methotrexate[d] Retinoids[d] Phototherapy[d] TNF-α inhibitors[d]		
Level of care	Primary	Tertiary Refer to dermatologist	Tertiary Refer to dermatologist

[d]Refer to dermatologist

Clinial features: Irregular, vitiligo-like areas of depigmentation are seen overlying bony prominences and are often surrounded by brown to blue-gray hyperpigmentation. Atrophy, xerosis and alopecia may be evident. Symmetric hypomelanotic macules enlarge until an entire area is affected. The most common sites are the dorsal aspects of the wrists and hands and over the metacarpophalangeal and interphalangeal joints.

Bejel

Hypomelanosis may occur in the late stages of bejel (endemic syphilis). Hypomelanotic macules have well-defined borders and may be admixed with pigmented macules. The lesions are usually symmetrically distributed on the extremities, genitalia, areolae and trunk. Early penicillin G treatment results in satisfactory repigmentation.

Syphilis

In secondary syphilis, hypomelanosis is an occasional finding that is called "leukoderma syphiliticum". In the "necklace of Venus", small (1–2 mm) hypomelanotic macules are scattered within a larger area of hyperpigmentation on the neck. Hypopigmentation may also develop at sites of previous inflamed lesions, which favor the neck, proximal extremities, upper trunk, abdomen, axillae and groin. Leukoderma syphiliticum regresses with treatment and usually disappears.

2. Onchocerciasis

Initially, small (punctate), yellow-brown hypomelanotic macules appear on the middle third of the shin medial to the tibial crest. Later, the macules enlarge, coalesce and undergo progressive lightening until there is amelanosis. Pigmented macules persist within the hypopigmented patches, hence the designation "leopard skin".

3. Post-kala-azar Dermal Leishmaniasis

Small hypomelanotic macules in a symmetric distribution that favor the upper trunk and arms constitute the prenodular stage of the disease. The lesions become elevated over a period of months to years. Total repigmentation following systemic treatment with antimonials is almost impossible to achieve.

Herpes Zoster

Hypo- or depigmentation is sometimes seen in the sites of previous herpes zoster. Amelanosis can result from melanocyte destruction during the inflammatory and healing process, which may also lead to atrophy and fibrosis.

CHEMICAL LEUCODERMA

A large number of chemical and pharmaco-logic agents can cause hypomelanosis of skin and hair. The major groups of depigmenting compounds are:

1. Hydroquinone (HQ) and its derivatives (MMEH, MBEH) are the most widely used "bleaching" agents. HQ induces a reversible hypopigmentation of the skin, and it is used to treat disorders such as melasma. In contrast, depigmentation from MBEH is often permanent and occurs not only in the areas of application but also in distant sites; as a result, its only indication is as depigmentation therapy for widespread vitiligo. In people who work with rubber, the same chemical can lead to occupational leukoderma.

2. Steroid abuse is another common cause. Hypomelanosis can follow the use of either topical or intralesional corticoste-roids, particularly in darkly pigmented individuals. In India, potent topical corti-costeroids are unfortunately widely used as lightening agents and in these cases the hypomelanosis is incomplete. A very common condition is hypomelanosis induced by intralesional or intra-articular corticosteroids.

MISCELLANEOUS LEUKODERMAS

Woronoff's ring: This is a blanched halo of fairly uniform width surrounding psoriatic lesions after phototherapy or topical treatments. The cause is presumed to be vasoconstriction.

Nevus anemicus: This presents as a pale area of variable size (often 3–6 cm) with an irregular, "broken up" outline (Fig. 2.26). It is usually unilateral, seen on the trunk and is most noticeable when there is surrounding vasodilation due to heat or emotional stress. On diascopy, the lesion becomes indistin-guishable from surrounding skin. It is believed to be due to decreased blood flow through the capillaries in the dermal papillae, and due to a localized hypersensitivity of the blood vessels to catecholamines.

> **Practice Pearl**
>
> In any patient, particularly adults, presenting with new-onset "vitiligo" a detailed history to detect exposure to known depigmenting agents is mandatory. Patch testing can be useful for confirming the diagnosis of chemical leukodermas, but delayed readings are essential (e.g. at 2 weeks, then again at 4–6 weeks). Spontaneous repigmen-tation may occur following avoidance of the causative agent, but treatment, as for vitiligo, is usually required.

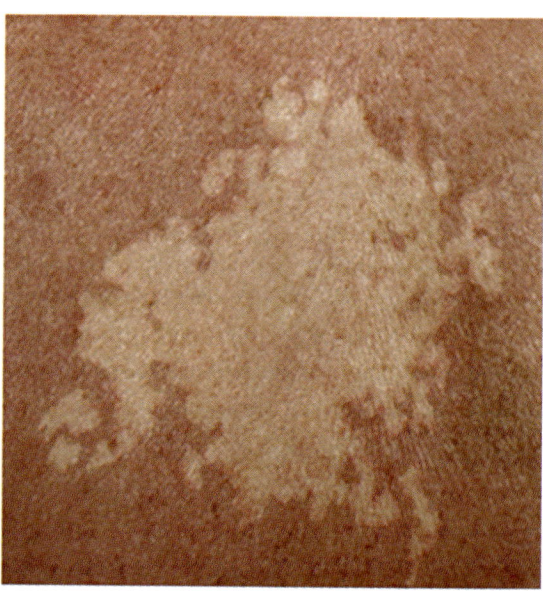

Fig. 2.26: Nevus anemicus

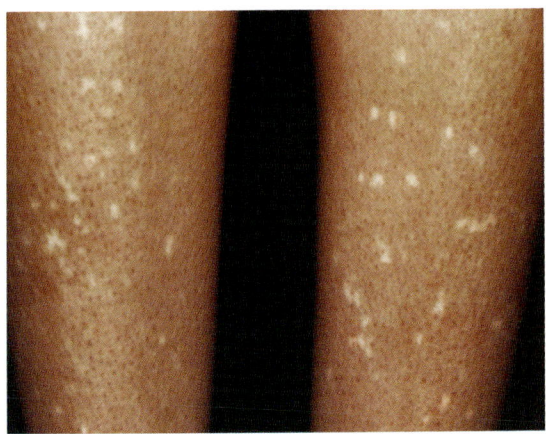

Fig. 2.27: Bier spots

Angiospastic macules (Bier spots): Pale macules, usually 3–6 mm in diameter, are seen on the extremities (often more noticeable on the legs) (Fig. 2.27). They are due to localized vasoconstriction and are seen most often in young women.

They can present with innumerable hypopigmented macular lesions with faint, irregular borders against blanching erythema in a mottled pattern over forearms and palms. Mottling is more marked over the palms. Their appearance may be induced by a dependent position or placing a tourniquet on the limb.

Bibliography

1. Badea I, Taylor M, Rosenberg A, Foldvari M. Pathogenesis and therapeutic approaches for improved topical treatment in localized scleroderma and systemic sclerosis. Rheumatology (Oxford). Mar 2009;48:213–21.
2. Breathnach SM. Rooks Textbook of Dermatology, 9th edn., Wiley Blackwell, United Kingdom, 2010.
3. Coelho-Macias V, Mendes-Bastos P, Assis-Pacheco F, Cardoso J. Imatinib: A novel treatment approach for generalized morphea. Int J Dermatol 2014;53(10):1299–302.
4. Cunningham BB, Landells ID, Langman C, Sailer DE, Paller AS. Topical calcipotriene for morphea/linear scleroderma. J Am Acad Dermatol. 1998; 39: 211–15.
5. Fett NM. Morphea: Evidence-based recommendations for treatment. Indian J Dermatol Venereol Leprol. Mar-Apr 2012;78(2):135–41.
6. Fett N. Scleroderma: Nomenclature, etiology, pathogenesis, prognosis and treatments: Facts and controversies. Clin Dermatol. 2013;31:432–7.
7. Goldsmith LA, Katz SI. Gilherst B, 2012, Fitzpatricks Dermatology in General Medicine, 8th edn., Mac Graw Hill education.
8. Ruffatti A, Peserico A, Rondinone R, et al. Prevalence and characteristics of anti-single-stranded DNA antibodies in localized scleroderma. Comparison with systemic lupus erythematosus. Arch Dermatol 1991;127: 1180–3.
9. Shiohara T, Kano Y, 2012, Dermatology, 3rd edn, Elsevier Saunders.

Disorders of Hyperpigmentation

Kabir Sardana, Pooja Arora Mrig

This chapter is subdivided for simplicity into common and rare disorders—linear and reticulate disorders. One important role of a primary care physician is to identify a problem and refer it to a specialist. Some of the disorders, like linear and reticulate pigmentation, fall in this category. We have provided tables of treatment, but it must be emphasized that specialized tests and interventions are not to be attempted by primary care physicians as they involve specialized skills and are fraught with medicolegal issues.

1. APPROACH TO HYPERPIGMENTATION DISORDERS

Hypermelanotic disorders present clinically with brown to slate gray colored macules. The color varies with the level of pigment deposition and also the type of pigment deposited. Hyperpigmentation is seen either as a consequence of increase in number of melanocytes, increased melanin synthesis, or deposition of nonmelanin pigment in the dermis. Disorders can be classified based on the age of onset, level of the pigment deposition and extent of involvement.

It is important to recognize that a few physiological conditions, like pregnancy, may be associated with increased pigmentation that is seen in 90% of women and is more common in darker skin types. The pigmentation becomes more intense in normally pigmented areas such as nipple, areolae, and genitalia. Pre-existing pigmented lesions become darker. Linea nigra is a median line seen over the anterior abdominal wall that is seen in pregnancy. Melasma has been seen in more than 50% of pregnant women. It is also called 'chloasma' or mask of 'pregnancy'.

Congenital conditions include Becker's melanosis and café au lait macules. Café au lait macules are coffee-colored lesions with well-defined borders that are associated with a variety of genodermatosis, the common among them are neurofibromatosis, tuberous sclerosis, McCune-Albright syndrome, etc. Becker's nevus is a hamartomatous condition presenting during adolescence. The lesion is a brownish-colored macule with geographical borders presenting over the shoulders, and upper chest. Overlying hypertrichosis and acneiform lesions are often seen. Associated extracutaneous anomalies include muscle hypoplasia, limb, and bone defects.

An approach to hyperpigmentation disorders is given in Flowchart 3.1.

Flowchart 3.1: Approach to diagnosis of common hyperpigmentation disorders

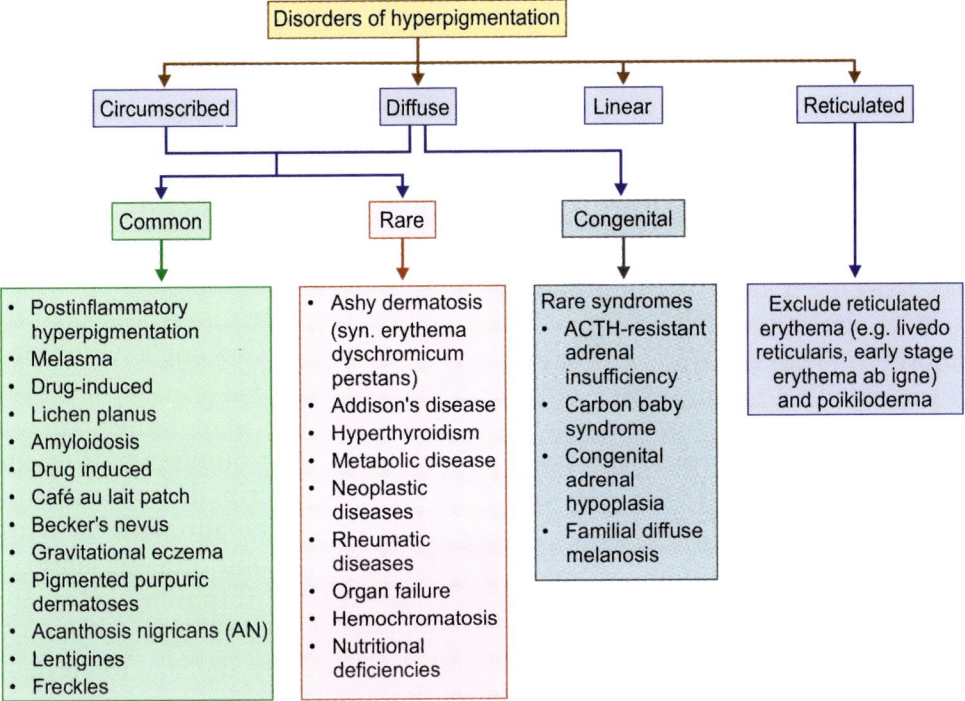

Facial hypermelanosis is a very common clinical entity seen in routine dermatological practice. It includes disorders such as melasma, Riehl's melanosis, poikiloderma of civatte, erythromelanosis follicularis, etc. Melasma is a common pigmentary disorder seen in females of reproductive age group. The etiological factors proposed include genetic predisposition, sun exposure, female sex hormones and intake of drug such as phenytoin and oral contraceptives. Lesions present over the convex areas of the face as hyperpigmented macules with well-defined borders. Another common cause of facial pigmentation is Riehl's melanosis also called pigmented contact dermatitis. The lesions present over the temples, preauricular area and neck as gray to brown-colored pigmentation in net-like pattern. The dermatitis is secondary to allergens present in kumkum, perfumes and cosmetics.

Poikiloderma of civatte presents clinically with brownish pigmentation, atrophy and telangiectasia present symmetrically on the sides of the neck and cheeks sparing the area under the chin. Histopathology shows solar elastosis with telangiectasia and melanophages in the dermis. This entity is often confused clinically with erythro-melanosis follicularis which presents with follicular papules on the background of pigmentation and telangiectasia in the preauricular area. Diagnosis is aided by histopathology which reveals lamellar horny masses in the sebaceous glands and hair follicles.

Dermal pigmentation presents clinically with bluish gray hue due to presence of melanin in the dermis. Common disorders included in this category are congenital conditions such as nevus of Ota, Mongolian spots and acquired conditions such as lichen planus pigmentosus, lichen planus actinicus, erythema dyschromicum perstans. Mongolian spots are bluish-colored macules seen most commonly in the lumbosacral area at birth. The lesions fade by 10 years of age or may even persist in adulthood. Nevus of Ota, also called nevus fusco-ceruleus ophthalmo-maxillaris, is seen commonly in females. It presents in young adults with bluish to brown-colored macules distributed along the ophthalmic division of the trigeminal nerve. The pigmentation is reticulate and associated scleral involvement is common.

Lichen planus pigmentosus is an acquired dermatosis presenting with slate gray to brown-colored macules distributed over photoexposed areas and flexures. The lesions are often asymptomatic to mildly itchy. Histopathology reveals basal layer vacuolization and lichenoid infiltrate in the dermis. Erythema dyschromicum perstans also presents with grayish coin-shaped macules with an inflammatory border present around the initial lesions. Etiological factors implicated in the pathogenesis include exposure to ammonium nitrate, radiocontrast agents, whipworm infection and HIV. The lesions appear first over the photoprotected sites. Differentiation from lichen planus pigmentosus can be difficult. Actinic lichen planus is a variant of lichen planus that presents clinically with viola-ceous plaques with perilesional halo on the photoexposed parts such as temples, preauri-cular area and neck. Coexistent lesions of classical lichen planus are seen in 20% of cases.

Another common entity seen in clinical practice that presents with slate gray-colored fixed recurrent macules is fixed drug eruption. Commonly implicated drugs are barbiturates and sulfonamides. Lesions are seen commonly on the lips, genitalia and acral parts.

Addisonian pigmentation is a pattern of pigmentation that is seen with a number of conditions. The pigmentation involves exposed areas, flexures, palmar and plantar creases, pressure-prone sites, increased pigmentation of normally pigmented sites such as nipples and genitalia, pigmentation of mucous membrane (buccal, gingival, conjunctival and vaginal), and linear nail streaks. Common disorders that cause such pigmentation include Addisonian disease, AIDS, cirrhosis, Cushing's syndrome, pheo-chromocytoma, etc.

Drug-induced skin pigmentation is seen commonly with numerous drugs that are routinely prescribed. These compounds stimulate the melanocytes to synthesize melanin, form stable drug–melanin complex in the dermis impairing clearance by macrophages, themselves get deposited in the dermis, cause damage to dermal blood vessels causing iron deposition and lastly cause post-inflammatory pigmentation. Drugs implicated with such pigmentary changes are antimalarials, amiodarone, cytotoxic drugs, minocycline, tricyclic antidepressants, and anticonvulsants. Sun-exposed parts and mucous membrane are the commonly involved sites.

Other rare causes of generalized pigmen-tation include hemochromatosis, nutritional disorders such as pellagra, sprue, vitamin B_{12} deficiency.

Bibliography

1. Dereure O. Drug-induced skin pigmentation. Am J Clin Dermatol 2001;2(4):253–62.

2. Kang WH, Yoon KH, Lee ES, et al. Melasma: Histopathological characteristics in 56 Korean patients. Br J Dermatol 2002;146(2): 228–37.

3. Nordlund JJ, Ortonne JP, Cestari T, et al. Confusions about color: Formulating a more precise lexicon for pigmentation, pigmentary disorders and abnormalities of "chromatics". J Am Acad Dermatol 2006; 54(5 Suppl 2): S291–7.

2. COMMON HYPERMELANOTIC DISORDERS

LICHEN PLANUS (LP)

This condition is diagnosed by the flat topped, shiny, papular eruption (Fig. 3.1). It is thought to be an immunologically mediated disease, though there may be a genetic susceptibility.

Clinical Features

The characteristic lesion of primary LP is a small, polygonal-shaped violaceous flat-topped papule (Fig. 3.1a). Surface is shiny and a network of fine white lines called Wickham's striae can be seen. LP is usually pruritic and can be associated with Koebner phenomenon.

The "seven Ps" of LP include:

1. Lesions are often *pruritic*, but they may be asymptomatic.
2. Lesions are often *purple* (actually red to violet).
3. Lesions tend to be *planar* (flat-topped) (Fig. 3.1a).
4. Lesions form *papules or plaques*.
5. Lesions may be *polygonal* (Fig. 3.1a).
6. Lesions may be *polymorphic* in shape and configuration—that is, oval, annular, linear, confluent (plaque-like), large, and small, even on the same person.
7. Lesions tend to heal with residual *post-inflammatory hyperpigmentation*, leaving darkly pigmented macules in their wake (Fig. 3.1b).

Most frequently involved sites are flexor surface of wrist and forearms, dorsal surface of hands (Fig. 3.2), anterior aspect of the lower legs (Fig. 3.3), neck and presacral area. Mucous membrane especially oral mucosa is involved in more than half of the patients (Fig. 3.4). Lesions are also present over glans

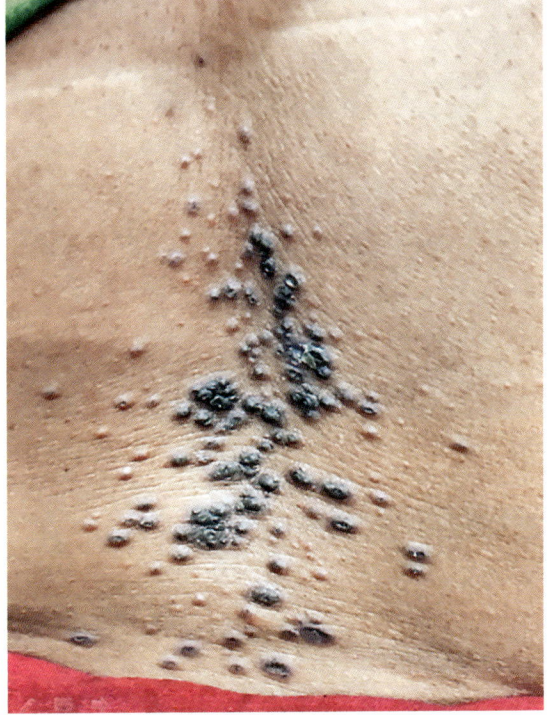

Fig. 3.1a: A 50-year-old female with pruritic polygonal violaceous papules over back suggestive of lichen planus

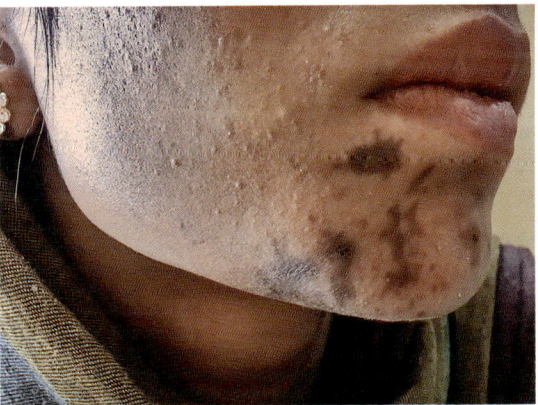

Fig. 3.1b: Residual pigmentation following lichen planus

where they can become erosive. Scalp involvement can lead to permanent hair loss (Fig. 3.5).

Other distinctive variants of LP include:

LP pigmentosus: A pigmentary disorder associated with macular pigmentation on

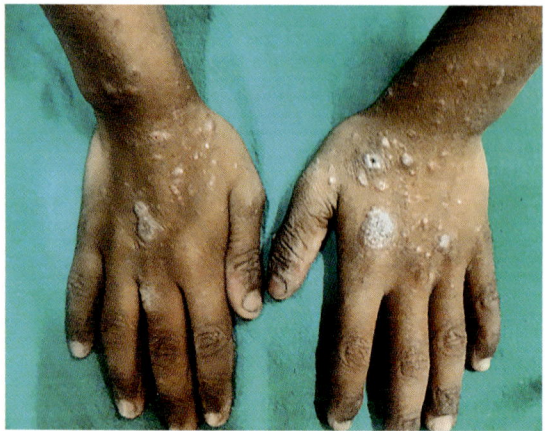

Fig. 3.2: Multiple, itchy papules on bilateral hands in a case of lichen planus

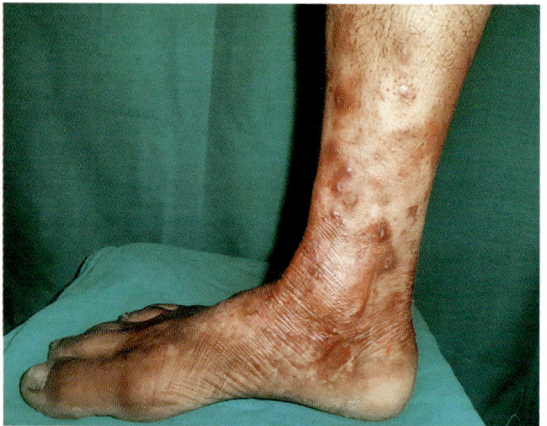

Fig. 3.3: A case of lichen planus on the lower limb. Note the pigmentary loss of the normal skin due to application of super potent steroid

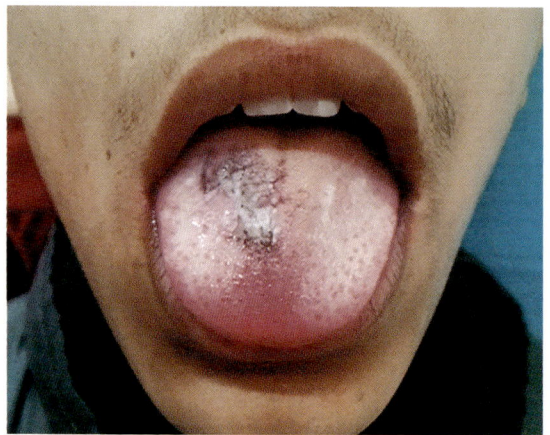

Fig. 3.4: A violaceous plaque in the mouth with 'Wickham's striae' (oral lichen planus)

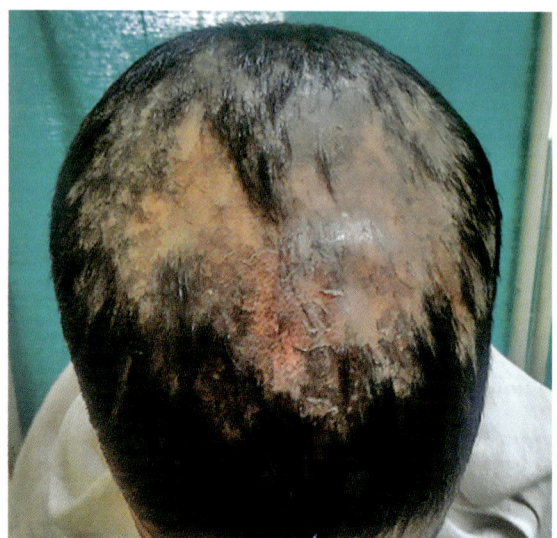

Fig. 3.5: Multiple follicular papules on the scalp (lichen planopilaris)

cheeks, face, neck, and upper limbs. It is slate gray to brownish black. Mucous membranes are not involved. (This is discussed in the section of Facial Melanosis.)

Other variants include: Actinic LP, guttate LP, nail LP, oral LP, ulcerative LP, vulvovaginal LP and drug-induced LP.

Investigations

- Histopathologic examination is characteristic in a biopsy of well-formed papule. Primary features are hyperkeratosis, focal increase in granular layer, irregular acanthosis with saw toothing appearance, liquefactive degeneration of basal layer and a band-like lymphocytic infiltrate at dermoepidermal junction. Colloid bodies and Max Joseph space can also be a feature.
- Direct immunofluorescence shows IgM and fibrin deposition at the dermoepidermal junction.

Diagnosis

It is based on clinical examination and characteristic histopathologic changes.

Treatment

LP is a self-limited disease that usually resolves over a period of a few months to one year. Mild cases can be treated with fluorinated topical steroids. Severe cases, especially those with scalp, nail, and mucous membrane involvement, require more intensive therapy.

Various therapies for LP include topical, intralesional and systemic corticosteroids, systemic retinoid, narrow band UVB, PUVA, topical calcineurin inhibitors, antimalarials, and for resistant, nonresponsive severe cases—oral immunosuppressive agents.

Topical Steroids

Steroids have anti-inflammatory properties and varied metabolic effects. Class I or II steroids in ointment form reduce pruritus in cutaneous lichen planus, but they have not been proven to induce remission.

Steroids in children: The adult and pediatric skin is different. Firstly, pediatric population has a larger skin surface area to body weight ratio. Secondly, their skin is thinner, which may result in greater amounts of topical steroid being absorbed compared with adults. Thus, milder steroids (Class 6/7) should be used.

Systemic Agents

Oral steroids: They are used in acute cases with severe involvement. The minimal daily effective dose for treating LP is 15–20 mg, for 2–6 weeks with gradual tapering doses.

Oral retinoids: Used in recalcitrant cases, dose of acitretin commonly used is 30 mg/day for around 8 weeks. As it is used in recalcitrant cases, relapses are common after discontinuation of therapy.

Oral cyclosporine has been used in cases non-responsive to oral steroids and retinoids. Mycophenolate mofetil can be used in disseminated, erosive, hypertrophic and bullous variants of LP.

Phototherapy. In cases of resistant long-standing LP, improvement has been observed with bath PUVA or systemic PUVA.

Table 3.1: Overview of treatment of LP			
	Medical management	*Cosmetic intervention*	*Laser/surgery*
Topical	Steroids Tacrolimus Pimecrolimus Intralesional steroids		Carbon dioxide, Nd:YAG laser
Systemic	Systemic steroids (30–80 mg/day) Retinoids[d] Cyclosporine[d] Mycophenolate mofetil[d] Dapsone Hydroxychloroquine Thalidomide[d] Azathioprine[d]		
Level of care	**Primary**	**Tertiary** Refer to dermatologist	**Tertiary** Refer to dermatologist

[d]Refer to dermatologist

Treatment of Oral LP

Good oral hygiene is important in management. Replacement of amalgam or gold dental restoration with composite material may improve the symptoms. Topical lignocaine gel can improve the symptoms.

Topical corticosteroids, such as triamcinolone, clobetasol propionate in orobase form, betamethasone mouthwashes or fluticasone propionate spray can be useful. Topical cyclosporine, tacrolimus or pimecrolimus can also be used for mucosal LP.

An overview of the treatment of LP is provided in Table 3.1.

Bibliography

1. Boyd AS, Nelder KH. Lichen Planus. J Am Acad Dermatol 1991; 25:593–619.
2. Breathnach S.M. (2010). Rooks Textbook of Dermatology, 8th edn., Wiley Blackwell, United Kingdom.
3. Cho BK, Sah D, Chawlek J, et al. Efficacy and safety of mycophenolate Mofetil for lichen planopilaris. J Am Acad Dermatol 2010; 62:393–7.
4. Goldsmith LA, Katz SI, Gilherst B (2012). Fitzpatricks Dermatology in General Medicine, 8th edn., Mac Graw Hill education.
5. Kanwar AJ, De D. Lichen planus in children. Indian J Dermatol Venereol Leprol 2010; 76:366–72.
6. Sharma A, Biaynicki-Birula R, Schwartz R A et al. Lichen planus: An update and review. Cutis 2012 Jul; 90(1): 17–23.
7. Shiohara T, Kano Y, 2012. Dermatology, 3rd edn., Elsevier Saunders.

POST-INFLAMMATORY HYPERPIGMENTATION

Post-inflammatory hyperpigmentation (PIH) is a common disorder that occurs in just about all individuals with skin of color and presents as residual macular hyperpigmentation that results from prior skin inflammation. This acquired pigmentation involves areas of prior inflammatory disease, infection, allergic contact or irritant reactions, injury from prior procedures or trauma, sites of papulosquamous or vesiculobullous disease, and medication reactions. It is more common in dark-skinned individuals.

Etiology

Various acute and chronic inflammatory skin conditions can lead to disruption of the basal layer of the epidermis leading to pigmentary incontinence and accumulation of melanophages in the dermis.

Clinical Features

History

The chief complaint of the patient with PIH includes dark marks, dark spots, uneven skin tone, discolorations, and blemishes (Figs 3.6 to 3.8). Patients with PIH have underlying cutaneous inflammatory conditions that may be clinical or subclinical or have a history of preceding trauma.

Physical Findings

The morphology of the macules and patches of PIH is variable, but the borders are often hazy and are distributed in areas of prior inflammation. When melanin is deposited in the epidermis, the lesions tend to be brown, but melanin in the dermis causes lesions to have a dark gray or gray-blue hue.

Treatment

Epidermal pigment may take 6–12 months to fade, whereas dermal pigment may be present for years. Underlying inflammatory conditions, if left untreated, could result in new areas of PIH.

There are several factors that influence the success of PIH treatment, including the location of the pigment, epidermal or dermal; adequate treatment of any underlying inflammatory disease affecting the skin; patient compliance; and the patient's response to available treatments. Resolution may be spontaneous, obviating the need for therapy.

Topical skin-lightening agents and physical modalities such as chemical peels, microderm abrasion, and laser treatments also may be used to treat PIH. However, these treatments may also induce hyperpigmentation owing to irritation and inflammation. Details about skin lightening agents are given in Chapter 7. Given below is a brief overview of these drugs.

Topical Drugs

1. **Hydroquinone:** Hydroquinone (HQ) has been considered the "gold standard" for treating all forms of hyperpigmentation. It prevents the conversion of tyrosine to dopa, in turn inhibiting the synthesis of melanin. Adverse events have been reported. HQ may induce irritation, erythema and scaling. Also in patients using HQ as a spot treatment, halo hypopigmentation may occur around the treated hyperpigmented patch. Additionally, exogenous ochronosis may also occur after long-term HQ use.

2. **Retinoids:** They may induce skin lightening owing to the epidermal melanin redistribution or dispersion. They also accelerate pigment loss by increasing the epidermal turnover and also inhibit tyrosinase enzyme. Retinoids may be used to treat various types of hyperpigmentation, including PIH. Tretinoin 0.1%, adapalene 0.1% gel, and tazarotene 0.1% cream all have demonstrated efficacy in improving PIH induced by acne vulgaris after 12–40 weeks of therapy. Recently, micronized and microsomal preparations have been launched which make the irritation of retinoids less. However, use of retinoids as monotherapy is not recommended for the treatment of hyperpigmentation due to their irritation potential which is likely to cause paradoxical hyperpigmentation secondary to inflammation.

3. **Azelaic acid and kojic acid:** The tyrosinase inhibitors azelaic acid and kojic acid also

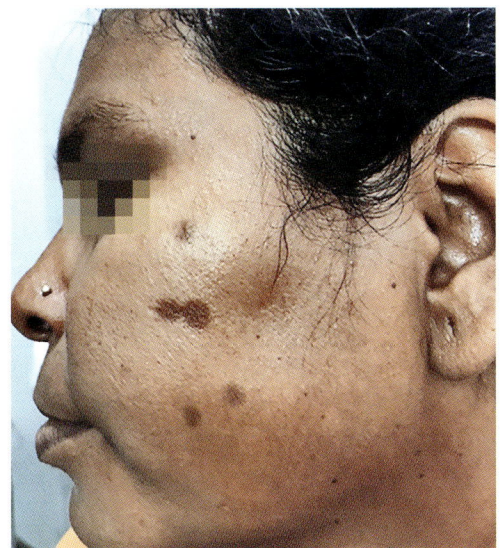

Fig. 3.6: Post-inflammatory hyperpigmentation over face secondary to spillage of hot oil

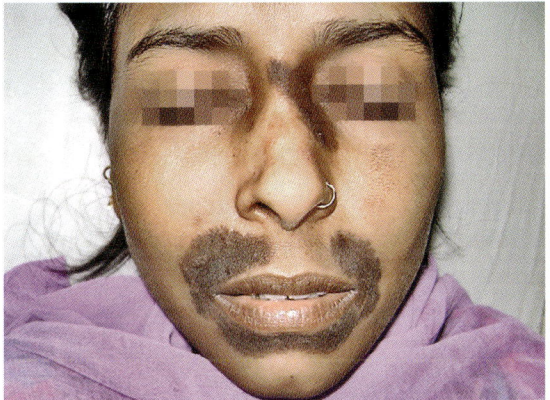

Fig. 3.7: A case of perioral dermatitis due to allergy to topical medication (nesoporin) leading to pigmentation

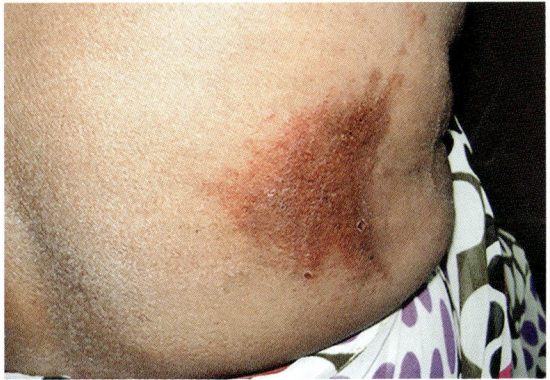

Fig. 3.8: A drug eruption (flagellate erythema) due to bleomycin, leading to pigmentation

	Medical management	Cosmetic intervention	Laser/surgery
Table 3.2: Overview of treatment of PIH			
Topical	Hydroquinone 2/4% Retinoids (tretinoin) Corticosteroids (mild/moderate) Azelaic acid Kojic acid **Combinations**[d] (Hydroquinone 4% + Tretinoin 0.05% + Fluocinolone Acetonide 0.01% or Mometasone furoate 0.1%) (Hydroquinone 4% + Retinol 0.15% + Antioxidants) (Hydroquinone 4% + Retinol 0.15%) **Non-HQ combinations*** Alpha Arbutin (0.5%) Niacinamide (2%) Glycolic acid (10%) Tocopherol acetate Tinosorb M (sunscreen)	Chemical peeling Salicylic acid > Glycolic acid (in Indian skin)	Lasers (not useful in Indian skin)
Systemic	Glutathione Tranexamic acid		
Level of care	**Primary**	**Tertiary** Refer to dermatologist	**Tertiary** Refer to dermatologist

[d]Refer to dermatologist, *Composition of a leading brand.

have been used in the treatment of PIH with varied efficacy and tolerability. They are generally considered second line therapy and are used in situations where HQ and/or retinoids cannot be used.

4. **Other non-HQ agents:** As HQ has been banned in Europe, a lot of compounds that mimic the action of HQ have been used. Some that are commonly used include, arbutin, niacinamide, and vitamin C/E, and 4-n-butylresorcinol. Various compounded preparations exist, some of them are detailed in Table 3.2.

Combinations

Recently, several combination therapies for PIH have been reported, including:

- Hydroquinone 4% and retinol 0.3%
- Mequinol 2% and tretinoin 0.01%
- Fluocinolone acetonide 0.01% and hydroquinone 4% and tretinoin 0.05%.

The last is called a triple combination (TC). It is important to understand that overuse of steroids can lead to side effects and thus while using these, the steroid component must be looked at. As a thumb rule, the order of safety depends on the steroid potency, thus the high potency to low potency steroids used in TC creams are, mometasone > Fluticasone > Fluocinolone acetonide > hydrocortisone. Thus, initially a TC with mometasone can be used but should be tapered down to safer and less potent steroids.

Cosmetic Treatments

Chemical peels, specifically glycolic acid peels, have been very helpful in the treatment of PIH. However, there is a risk of irritation to the skin and hence further hyperpigmentation. We prefer salicylic acid as it is safer, noninflammatory, suited for oily skin and also prevents acne, seen commonly in Indian patients.

Other treatments like, microderm abrasion alone or in addition to chemical peels have been effective in treating PIH, but in Indian skin may be counter-productive. Finally, various lasers, including the Q-switched ruby/Nd:YAG laser, fractional laser and the pulsed laser, have been used, although the adverse events outweigh the benefit of this form of therapy.

Bibliography

1. Amer M, Metwalli M. Topical hydroquinone in the treatment of some hyperpigmentary disorders. Int J Dermatol 1998; 37:449–450.

2. Griffiths CE, Finkel U, Ditre CM, Hamilton TA, Ellis CN, Voorhees JJ. Topical tretinoin (retinoic acid) improves melasma: A vehicle-controlled, clinical trial. Br J Dermatol 1993; 129: 415–421.

3. Grimes PE. A microsponge formulation of hydroquinone 4% and retinol in the treatment of melasma and post-inflammatory hyperpigmentation. Cutis 2004; 74: 362–368 2004; 74: 362–368.

4. Grimes PE. The safety and efficacy of salicylic acid chemical peels in darker racial-ethnic groups. Dermatol Surg 1999; 25: 18–22.

5. Javaheri SM, Handa S, Kaur I, Kumar B. Safety and efficacy of glycolic acid facial peel in Indian women with melasma. Int J Dermatol 2001; 40: 354–357.

6. Kakita LS, Lowe NJ. Azelaic acid and glycolic acid combination therapy for facial hyperpigmentation in darker-skinned patients: A clinical comparison with hydroquinone. Clin Ther 1998; 20:960–970.

7. Taylor SC, Torok H, Jones T, Lowe N, Rich P, Tschen E, et al. Efficacy and safety of a new triple-combination agent for the treatment of facial melasma. Cutis 2003; 72: 67–72.

PRIMARY (LOCALIZED) CUTANEOUS AMYLOIDOSIS

Macular and lichenoid forms of primary (localized) cutaneous amyloidosis are associated with hyperpigmentation. The most common locations are the upper back (macular amyloidosis) or the extensor surface of the lower extremities (lichen amyloidosis), where there is a characteristic rippled pattern (Fig. 3.9a and 3.9b) with parallel bands or ridges of hyperpigmentation. In nodular variant, there are nodules (Fig. 3.10). Areas of involvement are often pruritic, and rubbing plays a key role in the production of lesions. Histologically, melanophages as well as amyloid deposits that stain positively with antikeratin antibodies are seen within the upper dermis.

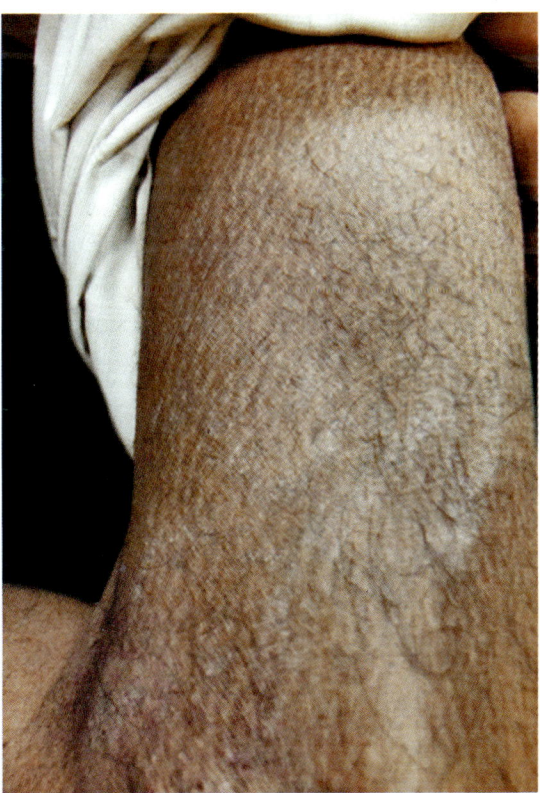

Fig. 3.9a: A patient with rippled pigmentation on the limbs (macular amyloidosis)

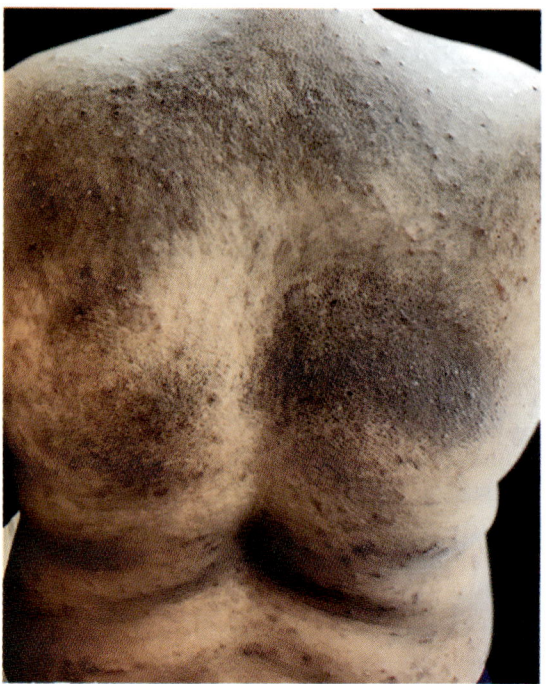

Fig. 3.9b: Extensive macular amyloidosis over back

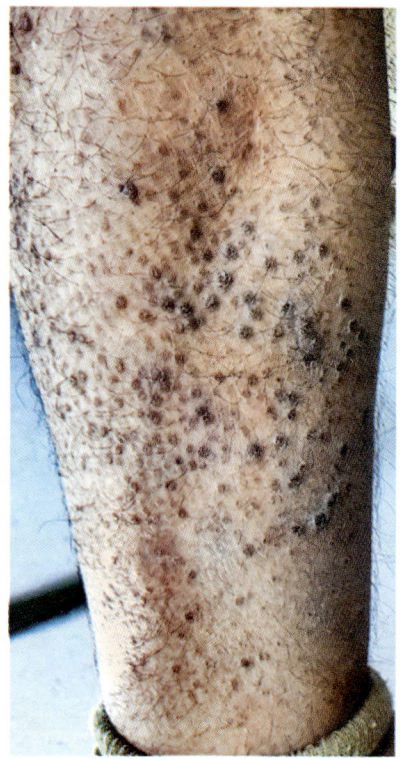

Fig. 3.10: A patient with severely itchy nodules on the lower limb (nodular amyloidosis)

Treatment

The condition requires a combination of topical steroids and systemic agents like colchicine, thalidomide, retinoids and PUVA. It is best to refer such cases to dermatologists.

Bibliography

Pigmentation Disorders. In: Sardana K, Garg VK, Mahajan S, eds. Diagnosis and Management of Skin Diseases: An Evidence Based Approach, Wolters Kluwer, LWW 2012, 1st edition.

DRUG-INDUCED HYPERPIGMENTATION

A wide range of medications (most commonly chemotherapeutic agents, antimalarials, minocycline, clofazamine and zidovudine) (Fig. 3.11a to 3.11c) and chemicals can lead to cutaneous hypermelanosis or discoloration (Table 3.3). The underlying mechanisms vary from induction of melanin production to deposition of drug complexes or heavy metals within the dermis. The pigmentation can be circumscribed or generalized.

Treatment

Although it usually resolves with discontinuation of the offending drug, the course may be prolonged.

- **Arsenic:** Areas of bronze hyperpigmentation ± superimposed "raindrops" of lightly pigmented skin; favors axillae, groin, palms, soles, nipples, and pressure points. It appears 1–20 years after arsenic exposure, with a strong dose-response relationship.
- **Chloroquine, hydroxychloroquine:** Gray to blue-black pigment, usually pretibial, with (hydroxy) chloroquine; face, hard palate, sclerae and subungual areas may be involved (25% of cases).
- **Clofazimine:** Diffuse red to red-brown discoloration of skin, conjunctivae (Fig. 3.11c).
- **Cyclophosphamide:** Diffuse hyperpigmentation of the skin and mucous

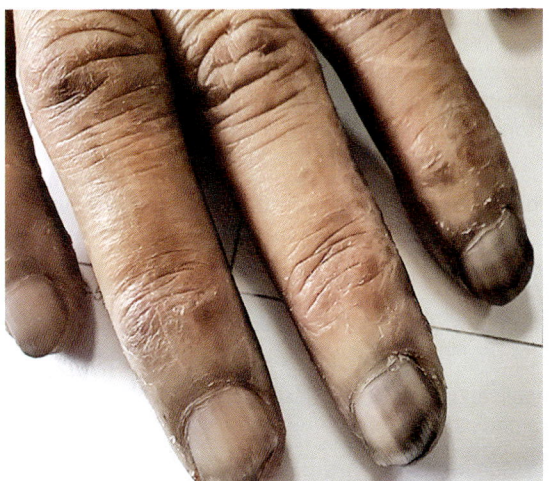

Fig. 3.11a: A PLHA on zidovudine (AZT). Note the characteristic pigmented band on the nails

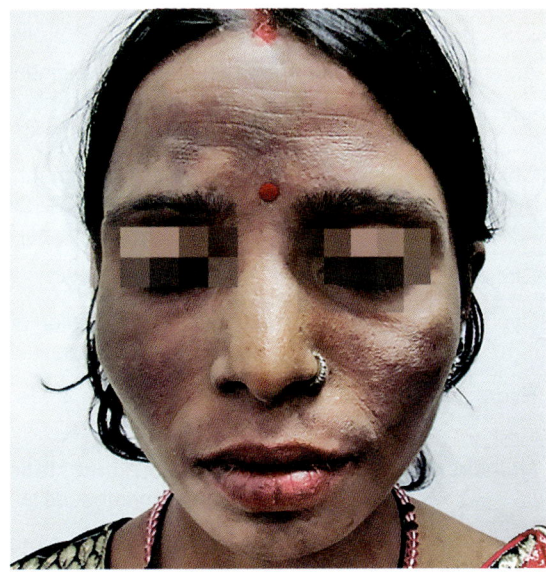

Fig. 3.11c: Clofazimine-induced hyperpigmentation over the face in a patient on multibacillary drug treatment (MDT) for lepromatous leprosy. Note the reddish brown color of pigmentation

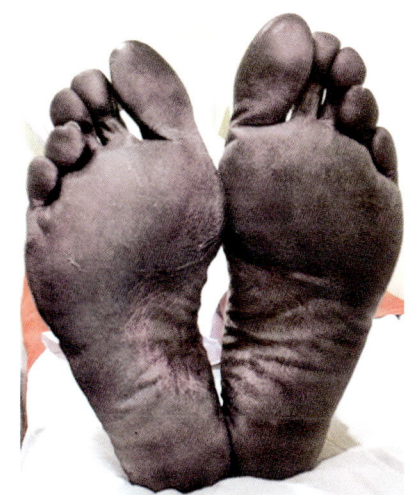

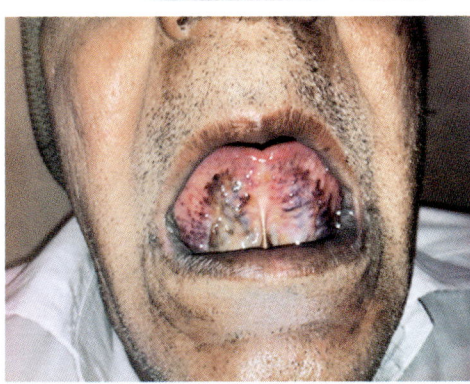

Fig. 3.11b: Chemotherapy (Epirubicin)-induced hyperpigmentation over soles and oral mucosa in a patient with adenocarcinoma of stomach. Similar pigmentation was present on the palms

membranes. Pigment localized to the nails (transverse, longitudinal or diffuse melanonychia), palms, and soles, or teeth.

- **Hydroquinone:** Hyperpigmentation in areas of application due to irritant contact dermatitis (i.e. post-inflammatory) or exogenous ochronosis.
- **Methotrexate:** Uniform hyperpigmentation in sun-exposed areas (occasionally follows an erythematous photosensitivity reaction).
- **Minocycline:** *Type I:* Blue-black discoloration in sites of inflammation and scars, including those due to acne. *Type II:* Blue-gray macules/patches (1 mm–10 cm in size) within previously normal skin, most often on the shins. *Type III:* Diffuse "muddy brown" pigmentation that is most prominent in sun-exposed areas. Blue-black discoloration may also involve nails, sclerae, oral mucosa, bones, thyroid and teeth.
- **Oral contraceptives:** Melasma; increased pigmentation of nipples and nevi

Table 3.3: An alphabetic list of drugs that commonly cause pigmentation

Arsenic	Areas of bronze hyperpigmentation ± superimposed "raindrops" of lightly pigmented skin; favors axillae, groin, palms, soles, nipples and pressure points. It appears 1–20 years after arsenic exposure, with a strong dose–response relationship (Fig. 3.11d and e)
Chloroquine, hydroxychloroquine	Gray to blue-black pigment, usually pretibial. With hydroxychloroquine, face, hard palate, sclerae and subungual areas may also be involved (25% of cases)
Clofazimine	Diffuse red to red-brown discoloration of skin, conjunctivae
Cyclophosphamide	Diffuse hyperpigmentation of the skin and mucous membranes. Pigment localized to the nails (transverse, longitudinal or diffuse melanonychia), palms and soles, or teeth
Hydroquinone	Hyperpigmentation in areas of application due to irritant contact dermatitis (i.e. post-inflammatory) or exogenous ochronosis
Methotrexate	Uniform hyperpigmentation in sun-exposed areas (occasionally follows an erythematous photosensitivity reaction)
Minocycline	**Type I:** Blue-black discoloration in sites of inflammation and scars, including those due to acne **Type II:** Blue-gray macules/patches (1 mm–10 cm in size) within previously normal skin, most often on the shins **Type III:** Diffuse "muddy brown" pigmentation that is most prominent in sun-exposed areas. Blue-black discoloration may also involve nails, sclerae, oral mucosa, bones, thyroid and teeth
Oral contraceptives	Melasma; increased pigmentation of nipples and nevi
Psoralens	Diffuse hyperpigmentation after exposure to UVA light following oral administration (PUVA)
Zidovudine	Longitudinal > transverse and diffuse melanonychia (up to 10% patients); blue lunulae Mucocutaneous hyperpigmentation (e.g. widespread diffuse, acral, oral macules); most common in patients with darkly pigmented skin, and may be accentuated in areas of friction or sun exposure

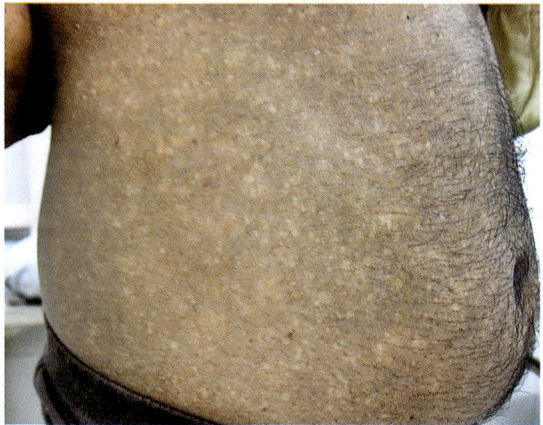

Fig. 3.11d: A patient showing mottled pigmentation with areas of hypopigmentation with a characteristic "raindrop" pigmentation due to arsenic intake via ayurvedic medicine for psoriasis

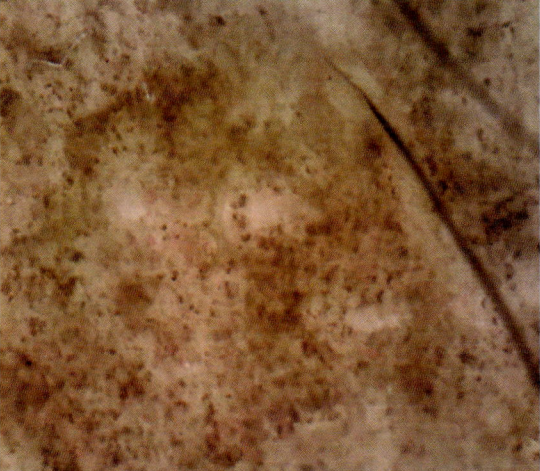

Fig. 3.11e: Leucomelanoderma seen in arsenic poisoning by using a dermatoscope

- **Psoralens:** Diffuse hyperpigmentation after exposure to UVA light following oral administration (PUVA).
- **Zidovudine:** Longitudinal > transverse and diffuse melanonychia (up to 10% of patients); blue lunulae. Mucocutaneous hyperpigmentation (e.g. widespread diffuse, acral, oral macules); most common in patients with darkly pigmented skin, and may be accentuated in areas of friction or sun exposure.

Bibliography

Pigmentation Disorders. In: Sardana K, Garg VK, Mahajan S, eds. Diagnosis and Management of Skin Diseases: An Evidence Based Approach, Wolters Kluwer, LWW 2012, 1st edition.

ERYTHEMA DYSCHROMICUM PERSTANS (SYN. ASHY DERMATOSIS)

This condition is often seen and possibly misdiagnosed as lichen planus pigmentosus though they possibly are manifestations of a similar spectrum. Ramirez first described erythema dyschromicum perstans (EDP) in 1957.

The etiology of EDP is not known. Although it has been postulated that a cell-mediated immune reaction to an ingestant, contactant or microorganism underlies the discrete areas of pigmentary incontinence, no causal agent has been consistently identified. In most patients, a trigger is never found. Various causes implicated include ammonium nitrate, oral X-ray contrast media, and medications (e.g. benzodiazepines, penicillin); exposure to various pesticides, fungicides or toxins; endocrinopathies such as thyroid disease; and whipworm and HIV infections.

Clinical Features

Oval, circular or irregularly shaped macules and patches that have a slate-gray to blue-brown color develop gradually in a symmetric

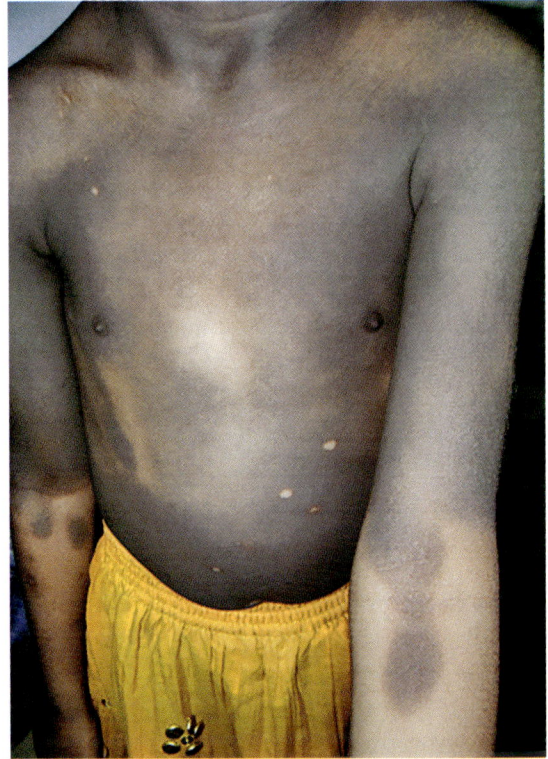

Fig. 3.12: Bluish macule on the trunk in a child with EDP

pattern (Fig. 3.12). The initial site of involvement is often the trunk, with subsequent spread to the neck, proximal upper extremities, and sometimes the face. The mucous membranes are spared, the palms, soles, and scalp are rarely affected. Occasionally, early stage lesions have a thin, raised, erythematous border, which tends to resolve over a few months, and the long axis of lesions may follow skin cleavage lines. Peripheral hypopigmentation may be seen in older lesions.

EDP is usually asymptomatic but can be mildly pruritic. The disease progresses slowly and usually does not regress in adults.

Treatment

There is no consistently effective therapy for EDP. Topical corticosteroids and hydroquinone are generally of no benefit.

Oralcorticosteroids, antibiotics, anti-malarials, isoniazid and griseofulvin, as well as UV light therapy, have produced variable results. Successful treatment with dapsone and clofazimine has been reported in small series.

It is best to refer such cases to a dermatologist.

Bibliography

1. Shwartz RA. Erythema dyschromicum perstans: The continuing enigma of Cinderella or ashy dermatosis. *Int J Dermatol* 2004;43:230–232.
2. Silverberg NB, Herz J, Wagner A, Paller AS. Erythema dyschromicum perstans in prepubertal children. *Pediatr Dermatol* 2003;20:398–403.

CAFÉ AU LAIT SPOT/MACULES (CALM)

Café au lait spots are uniformly pale-brown macules that vary in size from 0.5 to 20 cm and can be found on any cutaneous surface (Fig. 3.13a and b). They may be present at birth, are estimated to be present in 10 to 20% of normal children, and increase in number and size with age.

Six or more spots greater than 1.5 cm in diameter are presumptive evidence of neurofibromatosis (von Recklinghausen's disease) in young children over 5 years of age. In children under 5 years of age, five or more café au lait spots greater than 0.5 cm in diameter suggest the diagnosis of neurofibromatosis. Café au lait macules occur as solitary lesions in 10–15% of the normal population. Café au lait spots are present in 90 to 100% of patients with von Recklinghausen's disease. Smaller spots 1 to 4 mm in diameter in the axillae (axillary freckling or Crowe's sign) are a rare but diagnostic sign of neurofibromatosis. There is no increased incidence of café au lait spots in tuberous sclerosis.

Lesions that are similar but that have a more irregular border (shaped like "the coast of Maine") are seen in polyostotic fibrous dysplasia (Albright's syndrome).

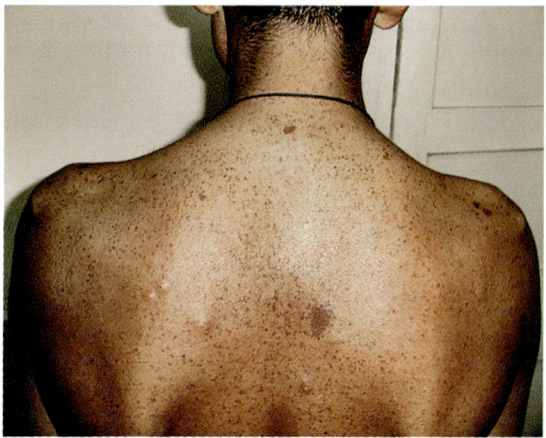

Fig. 3.13a: A case of neurofibromatosis with multiple brown CALMs and lentigines

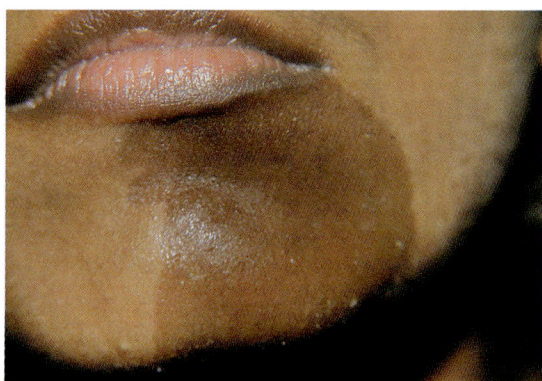

Fig. 3.13b: A single CALM on the face in a patient with no underlying disorder

The smooth, regular border of the café au lait macules of neurofibromatosis has been compared with "the coast of California".

Treatment

It is best to refer such cases as they require investigations to look for systemic associations. A few syndromes associated with CALMs are given Table 3.4.

Table 3.4: Syndromes associated with CALM
• Neurofibromatosis type 1
• McCune-Albright syndrome
• Bloom syndrome
• Watson syndrome
• Silver-Russell syndrome

MONGOLIAN SPOTS

Mongolian spots (MS) are non-blanchable hyperpigmented macules seen over the lumbosacral region in children at birth or in the first few weeks of life. These are prominent at the age of one and start fading after that.

They have a bluish green color with an oval or irregular shape. The blue color is due to dermal pigmentation secondary to dermal melanocytes causing a Tyndall effect. MS are most commonly seen in African and Asian populations.

Aberrant MS can occur over occiput, temple, mandibular area, shoulder and extremities.

Parents should be reassured that the lesions disappear with time. However, aberrant MS, size >10 cm, dark color and multiple patches are associated with persistence beyond 1 year. A few reports have suggested association between MS and inborn errors of metabolism.

BECKER'S NEVUS

Becker's nevus is a relatively common anomaly affecting 0.5% of young men.

Clinical Features

Site: Usually occurs in the scapular region. It can occur on other sites of the body like face, neck, and distal extremities.

It usually develops in adolescence as an irregular asymmetrical area of hyperpigmentation which may later thicken and develop coarse dark hairs (Fig. 3.14a to d). The prominence in adolescence with increased hair growth (hypertrichosis) shows that it is androgen dependent. It is more common in men. It may be associated with various anomalies, e.g. musculoskeletal abnormalities (scoliosis, ipsilateral limb hypoplasia), maxillofacial abnormalities, and cutaneous hypoplasias.

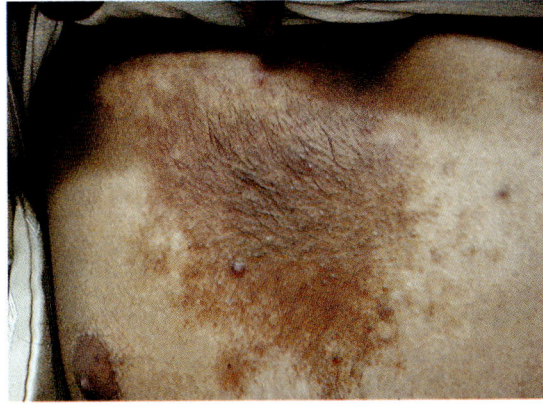
Fig. 3.14a: Becker's nevus

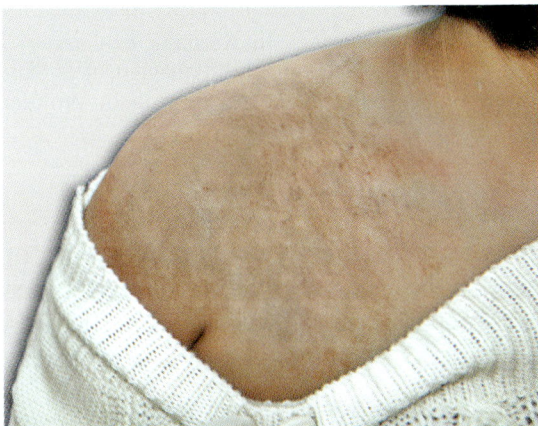
Fig. 3.14b: Becker's nevus in a young female patient

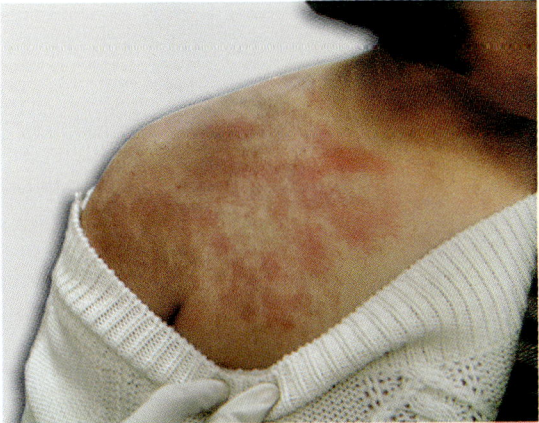
Fig. 3.14c: Becker's nevus following treatment with intense pulse light (IPL), note the immediate erythema

Becker's nevus remains indefinitely and can be treated with Q switched Nd:YAG or alexandrite laser (Fig. 3.14c and d).

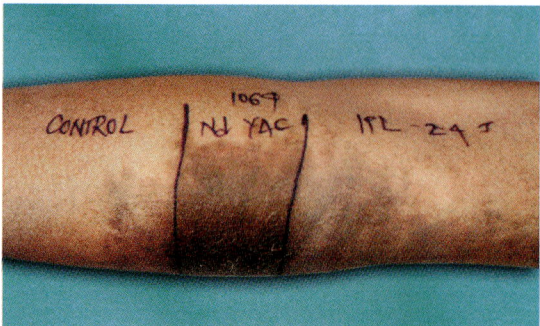

Fig. 3.14d: Becker's nevus on the limb, test spot with Nd:YAG (1064) and intense pulse light (IPL)

Bibliography

Pigmentation Disorders. In: Sardana K, Garg VK, Mahajan S, eds. Diagnosis and Management of Skin Diseases: An Evidence Based Approach, Wolters Kluwer, LWW 2012, 1st edition.

GRAVITATIONAL ECZEMA

Gravitational eczema is a common form of eczema that occurs on the lower extremities in patients with chronic venous insufficiency (Fig. 3.15a). It may be a precursor to more

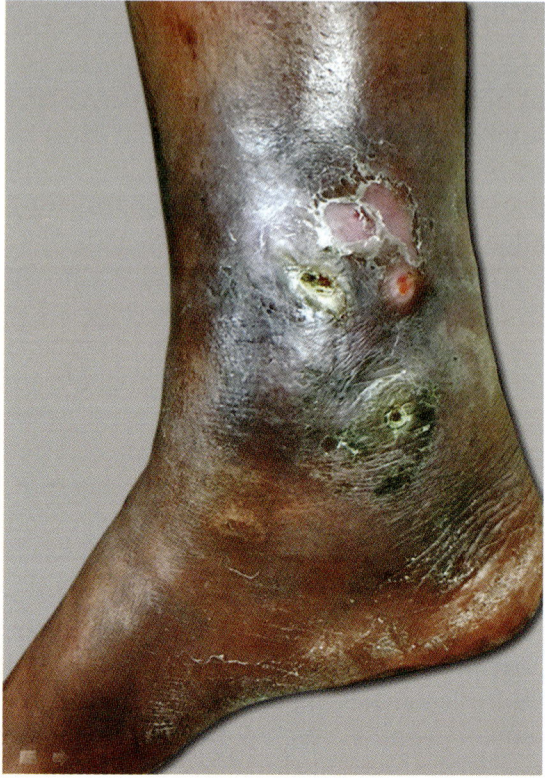

Fig. 3.15b: Hyperpigmentation secondary to stasis in an old male, labourer by occupation. Also seen are associated ulcers (venous ulcer)

problematic conditions, such as venous leg ulceration and lipodermatosclerosis or may be associated with ulcers (Fig. 3.15b).

Clinical Features

History

- Age: Adults and older patients.
- Itch is common.

Clinical Findings

- **Distribution:**
  - Localized or diffuse involvement of the gaiter area (Fig. 3.15a and b).
  - Often bilateral.
- **Morphology:**
  - Erythema
  - The skin may be dry and scaly, or weepy.

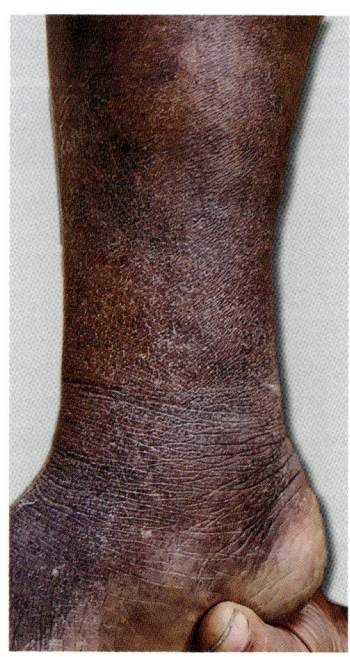

Fig. 3.15a: Diffuse pigmentation with edema in a case of stasis eczema

– A brown discoloration of the skin is common and results from hemosiderin deposition.

– Varicose veins may or may not be present.

Differential Diagnosis

Gravitational eczema is often misdiagnosed as cellulitis. Cellulitis is nearly always unilateral, tender and has a well-demarcated edge.

Treatment

Refer to a surgeon or dermatologist.

PIGMENTED PURPURIC DERMATOSES (SYN. CAPILLARITIS)

Progressive pigmented dermatoses (PPD) are characterized by petechiae and pigmented macules that occur symmetrically on the lower limbs. The condition, whose etiology is still unknown, is chronic and relapsing. There is extravasation of red blood cells and hemosiderin deposition in the skin. They have been divided into five clinical types with similar histopathological features:

• Progressive pigmented purpuric dermatosis (Schamberg's disease)
• Purpura annularis telangiectodes (Majocchi's disease)
• Pigmented purpuric lichenoid dermatosis
• Lichen aureus
• Itching purpura

Etiopathogenesis

The etiology is still unknown. Various cofactors that appear to influence the disease include venous hypertension and gravitational dependency, capillary fragility, exercise, infections, contact allergy, drugs, and chemical ingestion. Various drugs that have been known to cause PPD include acetaminophen, aspirin, chlordiazepoxide, reserpine, hydralazine, and interferon-alfa.

Recently, it has been postulated that cell-mediated immunity may play a role in pathogenesis of disease.

Clinical Features

We will focus on progressive pigmented purpuric dermatosis (Schamberg's disease) as this is the variant most commonly encountered in clinical practice.

It occurs most commonly in young adult males. The lesions are usually seen on the legs but may occur anywhere on the body. They consist of irregular plaques of orange or brown pigmentation (due to hemosiderin), with characteristic 'cayenne pepper' spots appearing within and at the edge of old lesions (Fig. 3.16). The condition is usually asymptomatic though slight itching may occur in a few patients. The eruptions are chronic and persistent and display slow proximal extension with some clearing of the original lesions.

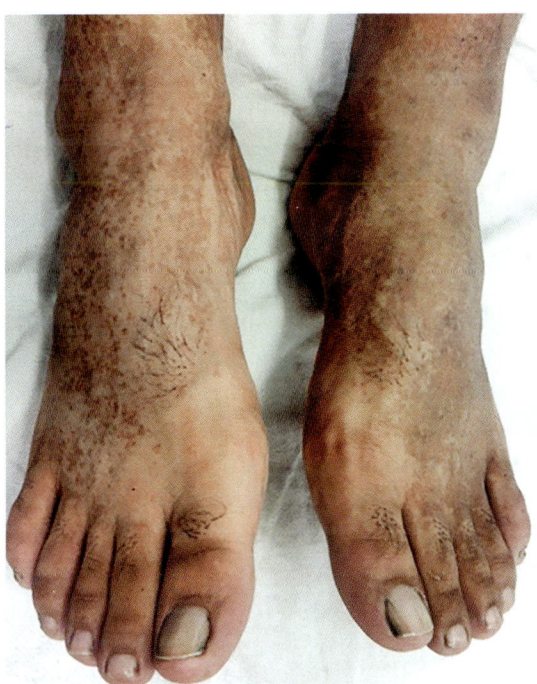

Fig. 3.16: Multiple pigmented macules on the lower limb in a case of PPD

Investigations

PPD is generally a clinical diagnosis and investigations are required only in doubtful or unusual cases.

Histopathology of skin shows perivascular infiltrate of lymphocytes and macrophages. There may be endothelial swelling and narrowing of lumina. The classical finding is extravasation of red blood cells with marked hemosiderin deposition in macrophages. Pearls stain and Fontana Masson help to demonstrate hemosiderin deposition in superficial dermis. Direct immunofluorescence reveals deposition of fibrinogen, IgM with or without C3 in superficial blood vessels.

Other investigations which can be done in doubtful cases include a full blood count with peripheral smear, coagulation screen (rule out other causes of purpura), antinuclear antibodies (ANA), rheumatoid factor (RF), anti-HbsAg antibody and anti-HCV antibody (to rule out systemic causes and associations).

Treatment

PPD are chronic and persistent, usually resistant to therapy. Withdrawal of suspected causes can help in some cases. Simple support hosiery can help in majority of cases that are associated with venous stasis. Prolonged standing should be avoided. Topical steroids can be used to control the itching.

Psoralen photochemotherapy has been found useful in a few studies. It alters the activity of the T lymphocytes and decreases interleukin-2 production. Other drugs that have been tried include griseofulvin (500–750 mg daily), pentoxyphylline (400 mg three times a day), cyclosporine, rutoside (50 mg twice daily) and ascorbic acid (500 mg daily).

An overview is given in Table 3.5.

Table 3.5: Treatment of PPD	
	Medical management
Topical	Steroid
Systemic	Antihistamines
	Psoralen photo-chemotherapy
	Griseofulvin
	Pentoxyfylline
	Calcium dobesilate
	Ascorbic acid
	Cyclosporine
	Rutoside
Level of care	Primary

Bibliography

1. Kwon SJ, Lee CW. Figurate purpuric eruptions on the trunk: Acetaminophen-induced rashes. J Dermatol 1998; 25:756–758.
2. Ratnam KV, Su WPD, Peters MS. Purpura simplex (inflammatory purpura without vasculitis). A clinico-pathologic study of 174 cases. J Am Acad Dermatol 1991; 25:642–647.
3. Smoller BR, Kamel OW. Pigmented purpuric eruptions: Immuno-pathologic studies. Supportive of a common immunophenotypes. J Cut Pathol 1991; 18:423–427.
4. Tristani-Firouzi P, Meadows KP, Vanderhooft S. Pigmented purpuric eruptions of childhood: A series of cases and review of literature. Pediatr Dermatol 2001; 18:299–304.
5. Wong WK, Ratnam KV. A report of two cases of pigmented purpuric dermatoses treated with PUVA therapy. Acta Derm Venereol 1991; 71:68–70.
6. Zvulunov A, Avinoach I, Hatskelzon L, et al. Pigmented purpuric dermatosis (Schamberg's purpura) in an infant. Dermatol Online J 1999; 5:2.

ACANTHOSIS NIGRICANS

The etiology of acanthosis nigricans (AN) is unknown. However, if the onset of lesions is rapid and the lesions are generalized, then malignancy must be suspected and an evaluation undertaken.

AN can be seen in a wide range of individuals, from those completely healthy as a normal variant to those with underlying medical conditions, although it is most often observed in darker pigmented individuals. AN is also believed to be a marker of endocrine disturbances, namely increased insulin secretion and insulin resistance. Therefore, the most common type of AN is associated with conditions with an elevated insulin blood level, such as in diabetes and obesity. There are many other possible causes of AN, including:

- Hypothyroidism
- Addison's disease
- Pituitary disorders

Medications associated with AN:

- Insulin
- Glucocorticoids
- Growth hormone
- Diethylstilbestrol
- Vitamin B₃ (niacin)
- Methyltestosterone
- Oral contraceptives.

Clinical Features

Classical acanthosis nigricans is characterized by symmetrical areas of verrucous, brown to black, velvety plaques, typically located on the posterior and lateral neck and axillae (Fig. 3.17a to c). Flexor surfaces of the extremities, inframammary folds and perianal area may also be affected. Rarely it may involve the dorsum of the hands. Interestingly, patients often refer to the appearance of the lesions as a 'dirty area', which they are known to vigorously scrub (Fig. 3.17).

Treatment

The mainstay of AN treatment is management of the underlying disease. If AN occurs as a result of obesity, weight loss is required. If malignancy is the underlying cause, successful surgery or chemotherapy will ameliorate AN.

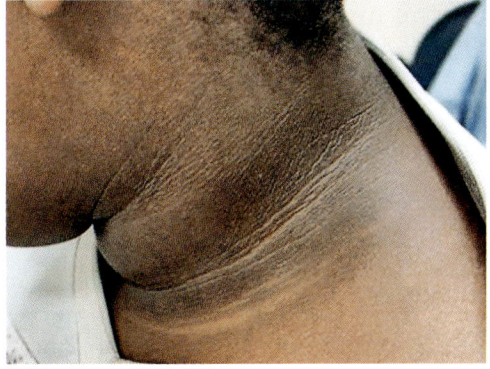

Fig. 3.17a: An obese individual with thickening of the skin with pigmentation of the neck (acanthosis nigricans)

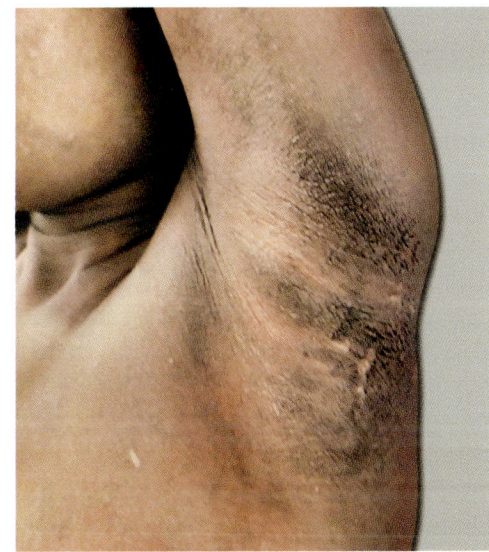

Fig. 3.17b: An 8-year-old boy with acanthosis nigricans over flexures. Work-up was normal and the condition was benign and idiopathic

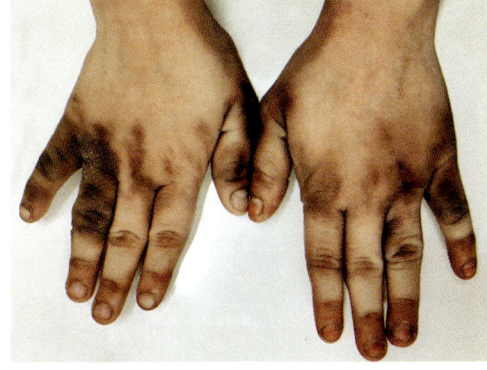

Fig. 3.17c: Acanthosis nigricans can rarely affect dorsa of hands

Topical treatments such as salicylic acid or tretinoin may be helpful in some individuals. Lasers or dermabrasion have also been used successfully, especially with verrucous protrusions. If AN is attributed to an offending agent, discontinuation of the drug should lead to resolution.

LENTIGINES

These lesions are persistent brown macules due to a linear increase in the number of melanocytes within the basal layer of the epidermis.

Lentigines may occur at any site on the skin, including the conjunctivae and mucocutaneous junctions (Fig. 3.18a).

Multiple lentigines are a common finding in people with fair skin, but may also rarely occur in rare hereditary multisystem disorders such as Peutz-Jeghers disease (particularly when distributed on the lips, buccal mucosae, and acral sites), centrofacial lentiginosis (associated with cardiac abnormalities), and the LEOPARD syndrome (i.e. lentigines, ECG abnormalities, ocular hypertelorism, pulmonary stenosis, abnormal genitalia, retarded growth, deafness).

Lentigines may also be caused by severe sunburn, especially on the upper back or

Table 3.6: Familial lentiginosis syndrome

- Carney complex
- Peutz-Jeghers syndrome (PJS)
- LEOPARD syndrome (lentigines, ECG conduction defects, ocular hypertelorism, pulmonary stenosis, abnormalities of genitalia, retardation of growth, sensorineural deafness)
- Arterial dissection and lentiginosis
- Laugier-Hunziker syndrome
- Familial benign lentiginosis
- Bannayan-Ruvalcaba-Riley syndrome (BRRS)
- Centrofacial lentiginosis
- Segmental lentiginosis

*Patients with lentigines and systemic abnormalities should be referred to a dermatologist for evaluation.

from chronic sun exposure (solar or actinic lentigines). They are common on the face and dorsal hands in middle-aged and elderly individuals (age spots or liver spots). Multiple solar lentigines may result from PUVA therapy or excessive sunbed use.

Syndromes associated with lentigines have been listed in Table 3.6.

Treatment

Prevention of further UV damage by sunavoidance and sunscreen use. Gentle cryotherapy and lasers (Fig. 3.18b) may be used to fade benign facial lentigines.

FRECKLES

Pale brown macules, less than 3 mm in diameter, due to the UV-induced production of melanin by a normal number of basal melanocytes. They are multiple and distributed on sun-exposed sites. Freckles are prominent during the summer, following UV exposure, and virtually disappear in the winter. They are very common, especially in children and individuals with type I or II skin.

Lentigines may be very similar in appearance but persist in the absence of UV stimulation.

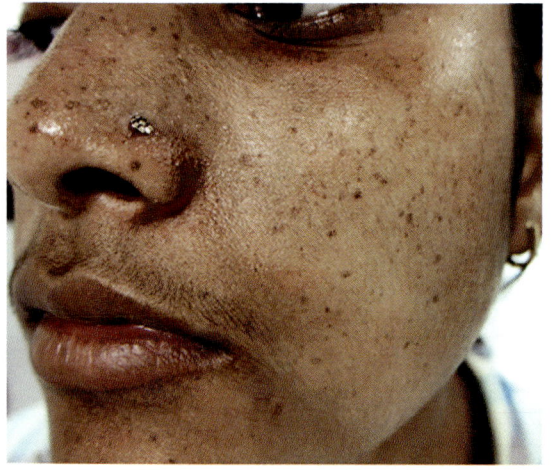

Fig. 3.18a: Multiple lentigines in a female

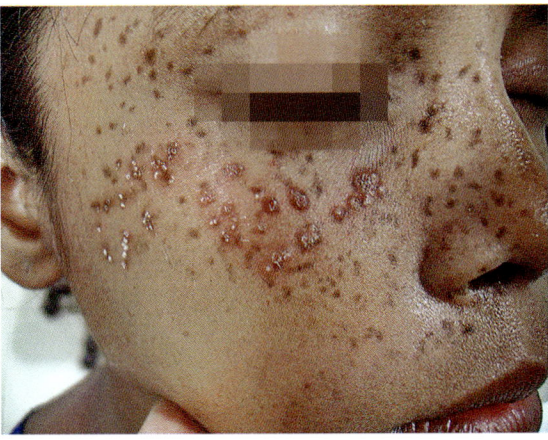 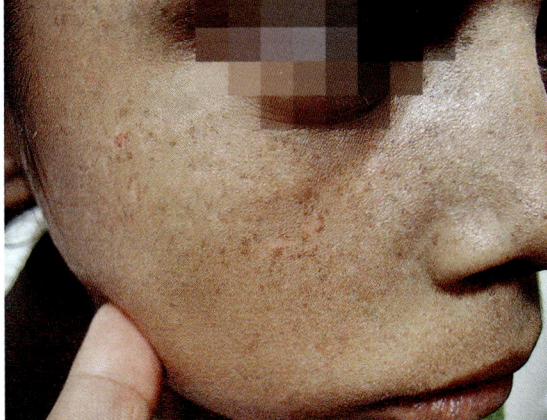

Fig. 3.18b: Patient being treated with Qs532 nm laser, note the immediate whitening of the lentigines (left), healing with reduction of lesions (right)

3. RARE DISORDERS OF HYPERPIGMENTATION

ADDISON'S DISEASE

Hyperpigmentation is a well-known feature of Addison's disease and occurs due to increased secretion of melanotropic hormones by the pituitary gland.

Clinical Features

Systemic Features

They include fatigue, weight loss, dizziness on standing, abdominal pain, vomiting and psychiatric symptoms.

Skin

Hyperpigmentation: There is diffuse hyperpigmentation with accentuation in sun-exposed sites, palmar creases, buccal mucosa, gums, scars, hair, nails and areas subject to friction. There is accentuation of normally pigmented areas such as the areolae, axillae, genital skin and umbilicus.

Investigations
- Low serum sodium and raised serum potassium.
- Serum urea and albumin are raised because of dehydration.

- Serum cortisol level taken ideally between 8–9 AM (random measurements have a low sensitivity for Addison's disease due to the pulsatile nature and diurnal variation of cortisol secretion). If the level of serum cortisol is:
  - <100 nmol/L—adrenal insufficiency is highly likely (if the patient is not on oral or inhaled steroids).
  - >400 nmol/L—adrenal insufficiency is unlikely (diagnosis not excluded if the patient is acutely unwell at the time since cortisol values may increase during illness).
  - Between 100 and 400 nmol/L—refer to a specialist for further investigations, e.g. ACTH stimulation test.

HYPERTHYROIDISM

Hyperpigmentation can occur in patients with hyperthyroidism and occurs due to increased secretion of ACTH from the pituitary in response to increase in the cortisol degradation. The pigmentation is diffuse and of Addisonian type. The classical Jellinek's sign (hyperpigmentation of eyelids) is seen in a few patients. Rarely, melasma-like pigmentation may occur.

HYPERPIGMENTATION IN NEOPLASTIC DISEASES

Hyperpigmentation is a variable feature of malignant tumors and may be seen in association with solid malignant tumors (oat cell carcinoma of the bronchus, malignant melanoma), pheochromocytoma, carcinoid syndrome and lymphomas. Secretion of ectopic ACTH (having MSH-like activity) or MSH analog is responsible in most of these cases (Fig. 3.19). Underlying genetic predisposition is seen in a few patients.

Hyperpigmentation can be diffuse or localized. The color can vary depending on the depth of pigmentation (epidermal or dermal). Non-melanin pigmentation can occur. Addisonian pigmentation is seen in ectopic ACTH syndrome (Fig. 3.19),

lymphomas and pheochromocytoma. Associated cutaneous features (e.g flushing in patients with carcinoid syndrome, diffuse slate gray dermal melanosis in malignant melanoma) can help in the diagnosis of the malignancy.

HYPERPIGMENTATION IN RHEUMATIC DISEASES

Scleroderma

It is an autoimmune disorder causing sclerosis in skin and internal organs like gastrointestinal tract, liver, lungs, and kidneys. The following patterns of hyperpigmentation can be seen:

- Diffuse pigmentation with accentuation in sun-exposed sites and areas of pressure (Fig. 3.20a).

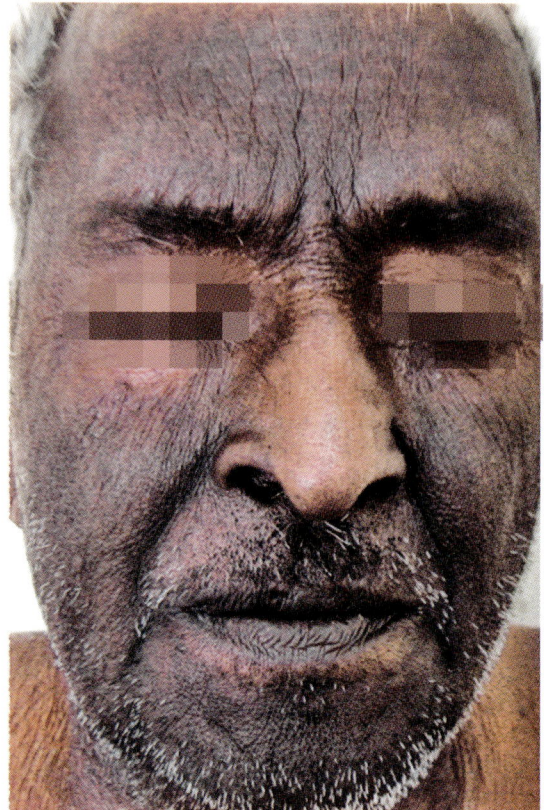
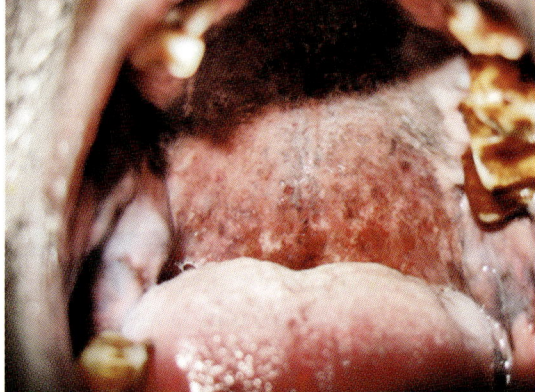
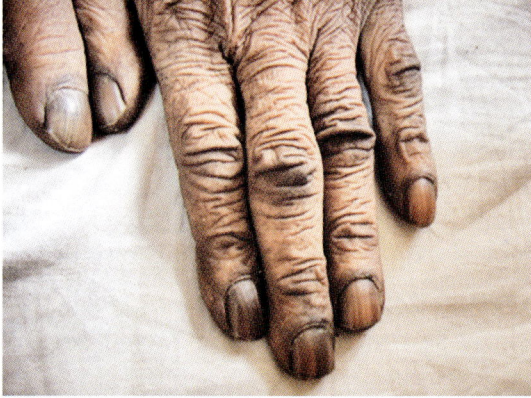

Fig. 3.19: Hyperpigmentation over the face, nails and oral mucosa in a 65-year-old male. Investigations revealed a small cell carcinoma of lung. Pigmentation was secondary to ectopic ACTH secretion by the tumor cells

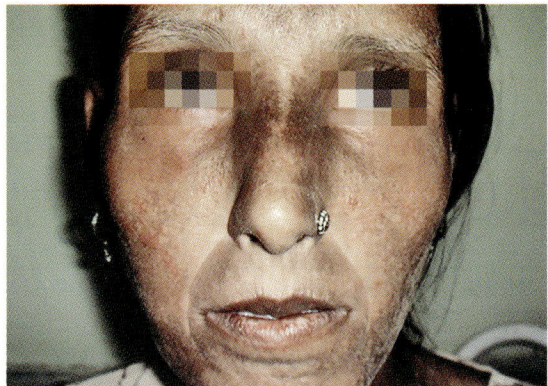

Fig. 3.20a: Melasma-like pigmentation in a case of scleroderma

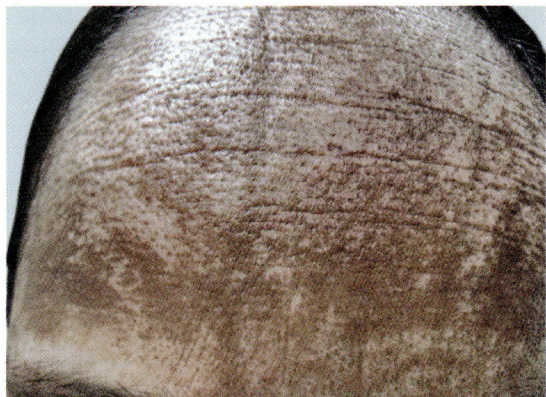

Fig. 3.20b: "Salt and pepper" pigmentation in a case of scleroderma

- Addisonian pigmentation
- Salt and pepper pigmentation with areas of hyper- and hypomelanosis (Fig. 3.20b).

Dermatomyositis and Lupus Erythematosus

Diffuse pigmentation may accompany the cutaneous eruption in these diseases and may be due to the disease *per se* or due to treatment with antimalarials.

HYPERPIGMENTATION DUE TO ORGAN FAILURE

Renal Failure

Increased pigmentation of skin may be seen in patients with chronic renal failure and is

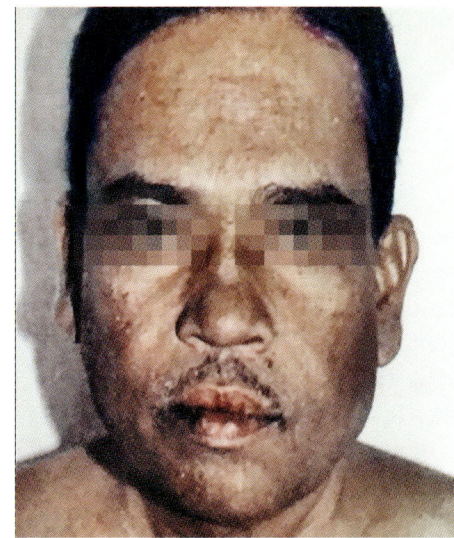

Fig. 3.21: Hyperpigmentation over the face in a male with chronic liver disease secondary to alcoholism (*Courtesy*: Dr Shikha Bansal)

largely due to elevated levels of β-MSH caused by slow clearance by the kidneys. Carotenoids and lipochromes may also be responsible for the phenomenon. It manifests as diffuse brownish pigmentation of body most pronounced in sun-exposed areas, especially the hands and face. Palms and soles may show hyperpigmented macules.

Primary Biliary Cirrhosis

Diffuse hyperpigmentation with accentuation in sun-exposed areas can be seen in patients with primary biliary cirrhosis and in alcoholic liver disease (Fig. 3.21).

HEMOCHROMATOSIS

Clinical Features

Systemic Features

Hemochromatosis results in diabetes, cirrhosis and cardiac failure.

Skin

Hyperpigmentation: Slate gray or brown-bronze with a predominance for the face and other UV-exposed sites.

Investigations

- *Iron levels:* Most people with hemochromatosis have elevated levels of iron in the blood.
- *Transferrin saturation:* Transferrin is a protein that binds iron and transports it between the tissues. This test is one of the most sensitive tests for detecting early hemochromatosis. A transferrin saturation greater than 45% should be investigated further.
- *Ferritin levels:* Ferritin is a protein that reflects the body's iron stores. Blood ferritin levels increase when the body's iron stores increase; however, levels of ferritin usually do not rise until iron stores are high. Therefore, ferritin levels may be normal early in the course of hemochromatosis. Ferritin levels greater than 400 ng/mL support a diagnosis of hemochromatosis, however, ferritin levels can also be increased in other conditions.

HYPERPIGMENTATION DUE TO NUTRITIONAL DEFICIENCIES

Nutritional deficiencies associated with hyperpigmentation are depicted in Table 3.7. Though except for pellagra and zinc deficiency the rest do not have a typical morphology.

4. LINEAR HYPERPIGMENTATION

There are multiple causes of a linear pigmentation including PDL (discussed later on), PIH and disorders along the lines of Blaschko. The Blaschko's lines are characterized by a V-shape on the posterior midline, an S-shape on the abdomen, and spirals on the posterior scalp. Dermatoses that follow the lines of Blaschko result from mosaicism. These are beyond the scope of the book and are best referred to dermatologists. A few pigmentary disorders that can present in a linear distribution are listed in Table 3.8.

LINEAR AND WHORLED NEVOID HYPERMELANOSIS (LWNH)

Linear and whorled nevoid hypermelanosis (LWNH) also called zosteriform hyperpigmentation.

In this condition, hyperpigmented macules occur in a streaky configuration along lines of Blaschko. There is no preceding inflammation or atrophy. Lesions occur over the trunk and extremities and do not cross the midline. The pigmentation decreases with age. It may be associated with extracutaneous abnormalities.

Table 3.7: Nutritional deficiencies and the associated cutaneous findings	
Disease	*Cutaneous manifestations*
Vitamin A deficiency	Generalized hyperpigmentation, hypermelanoses of face and extremities, associated dryness and scaling, conjunctival pigmentation, phrynoderma
Vitamin B_{12} deficiency	Dappled and mottled pigmentation of face and dorsa of hands and feet, rarely generalized, hyperpigmentation of mucosae, hypopigmentation of hair
Folate deficiency	Diffuse brown hyperpigmentation
Pellagra (vitamin B_3 deficiency)	Hyperpigmentation and cracking of skin of sun-exposed sites, mucosae may be affected
Vagabond's disease (poor diet, lack of hygiene, heavy lice infestation)	Addisonian pattern of hyperpigmentation, mucosae may be involved, hypomelanoses can occur

Table 3.8: Disorders associated with linear distribution of pigmentary lesions

Onset	Disorder
Congenital	Incontinentia pigmenti Verrucous epidermal nevus Linear and whorled hypermelanosis Nevoid linear hypermelanosis (Fig. 3.22a)
Acquired	Post-inflammatory hyperpigmentation secondary to herpes zoster, intravenous drug injection, dermatitis artefacta, pedrous dermatitis, and lichen planus (Fig. 3.22b) Pigmentary demarcation lines Aquired brachial cutaneous dyschromatosis (ABCD) (Fig. 3.22c)

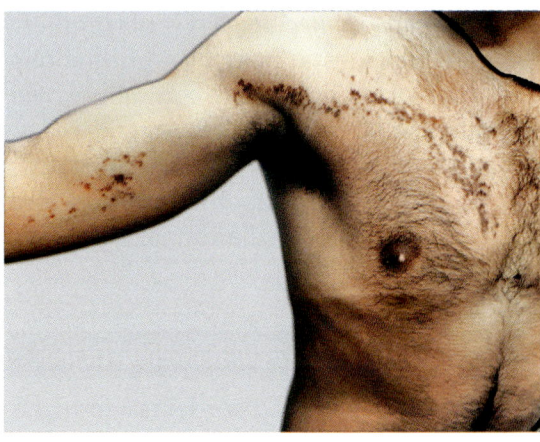

Fig. 3.22b: Linear lichen planus healing with hyperpigmented macules in a whorled streaky pattern on the trunk extending onto the extremity

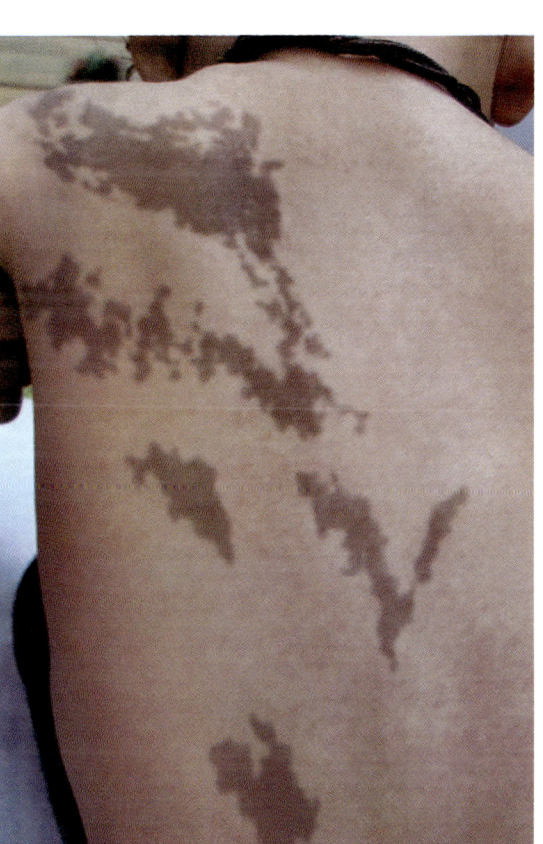

Fig. 3.22a: Linear pigmented macule on the back in a case of linear and whorled nevoid hypermelanosis

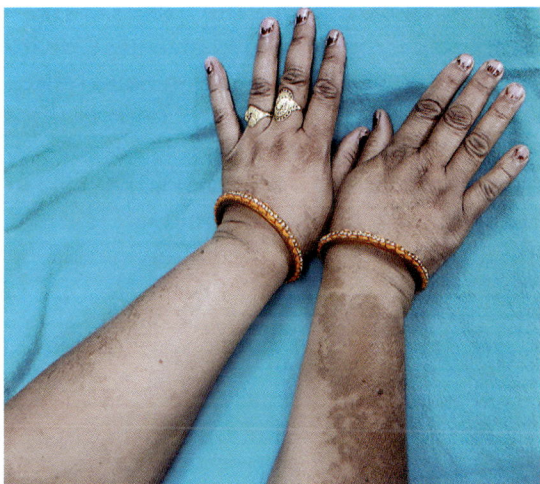

Fig. 3.22c: Brown patches with geographic border seen on lateral aspect of forearms

INCONTINENTIA PIGMENTI (IP)

It is an X-linked dominant disorder presenting in females. The condition is lethal in males in embryonic stage.

There are four stages of cutaneous involvement in IP.

1. *Vesicular stage:* It is seen from birth to shortly thereafter.
2. *Verrucous stage:* Verrucous lesions appear along lines of Blaschko between 2 and 8 weeks of age.

3. *Hyperpigmented stage:* Hyperpigmented macules appear in whorls along lines of Blaschko more commonly over the trunk. It fades after several years.

4. Linear atrophic hypopigmented scars occur along Blaschko's lines and represent post-inflammatory dermal scarring.

5. RETICULATE HYPERPIGMENTATION

Reticulate pigmentary disorder is a term, i.e. loosely defined to include a spectrum of acquired and congenital conditions with different morphologies.

The presentations vary from the reticular or net-like pattern to the "freckle-like" hyper- and hypopigmented macules that are usually restricted to the true genetic reticulate pigmentary disorders. There is little clarity on this topic and related terms, in major dermatology textbooks. Hence, to harmonize the different entities, we feel that the term "mottled pigmentation" could be used to include:

a. Reticulate pigmentary disorders (acquired and congenital), and

b. Dyschromatosis.

Dyschromatoses are characterized by the presence of both hypo- and hyperpigmentation (Fig. 3.23). Often, at least one component of the dyspigmentation is guttate.

A depiction of some entites is given in Fig. 3.24a and b. An overview is depicted in Flowchart 3.2.

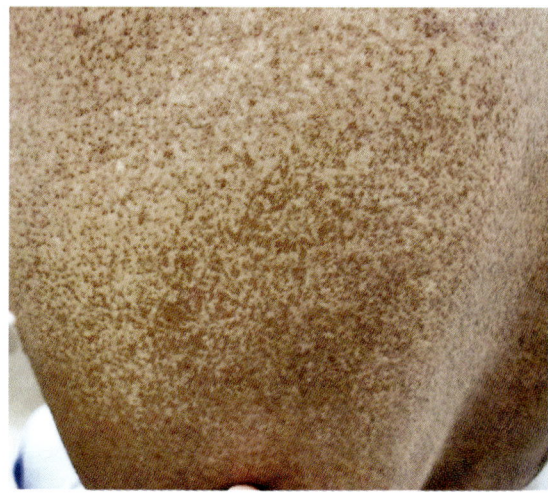

Fig. 3.23: Hypopigmented and hyperpigmented macules without atrophy (dyschromatosis universalis hereditaria)

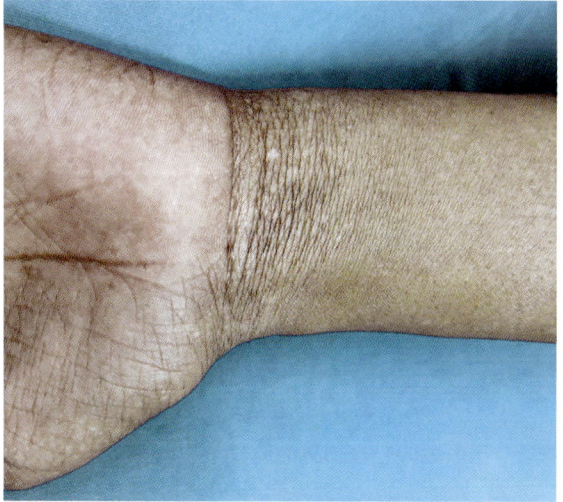 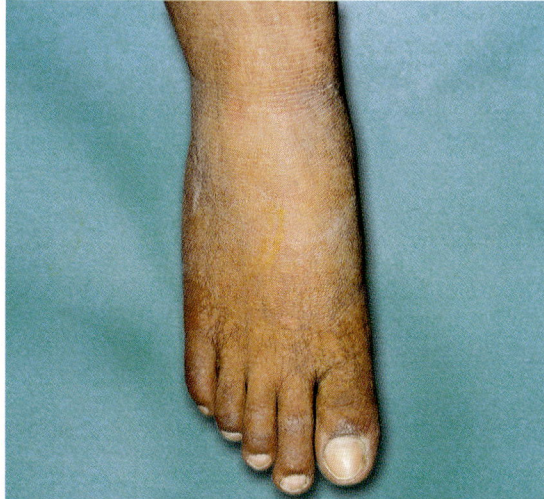

Fig. 3.24a and b: Reticulate pigmentation on the dorsal aspect of feet and hand in a case of reticulate pigmentation of Kitamura

Flowchart 3.2: Classification of reticulate pigmentation disorders

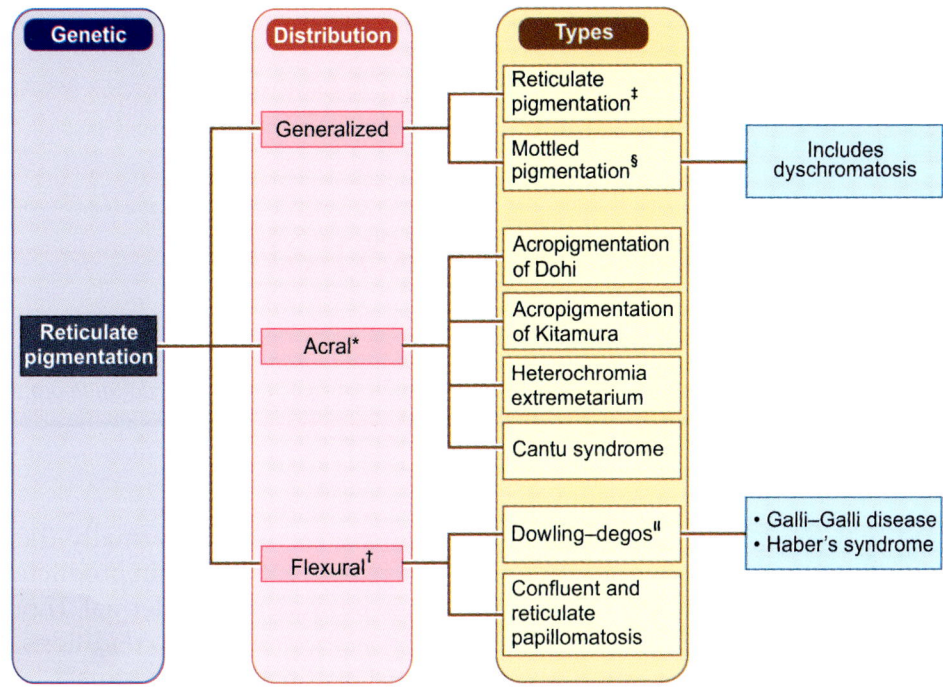

*Acromelanosis progressiva is another rare disorder.

†Rare: Anonychia with flexural pigmentation.

‡Dyskeratosis congenita, Fanconi anemia, X-linked reticulate pigmentary disorder, pachyonychia congenita, Mendes de Costa syndrome, Naegeli-Franceschetti-Jadassohn syndrome (NFJS), Berlins syndrome, Cantu syndrome, dermatopathia pigmentosa reticularis.

§Dyschromatosis universalis hereditaria, epidermolysis bullosa (EB) simplex with mottled pigmentation.

‖May be generalized later in life.

Facial Pigmentation

Kabir Sardana, Pooja Arora Mrig

It is said that the face is the passport to society. Consequently, pigmentation disorders of the face are of major concern in pigmented skins, more so in India, where there is fixation on fair skin with the face being the focus of attention. Facial hypermelanoses are a group of disorders characterized by abnormally darker skin due to increased melanin production which could be epidermal or dermal. Though there is an elaborate list of conditions, we will focus on the common causes. A simple flowchart is given to depict the commonly seen disorders (Fig. 4.1).

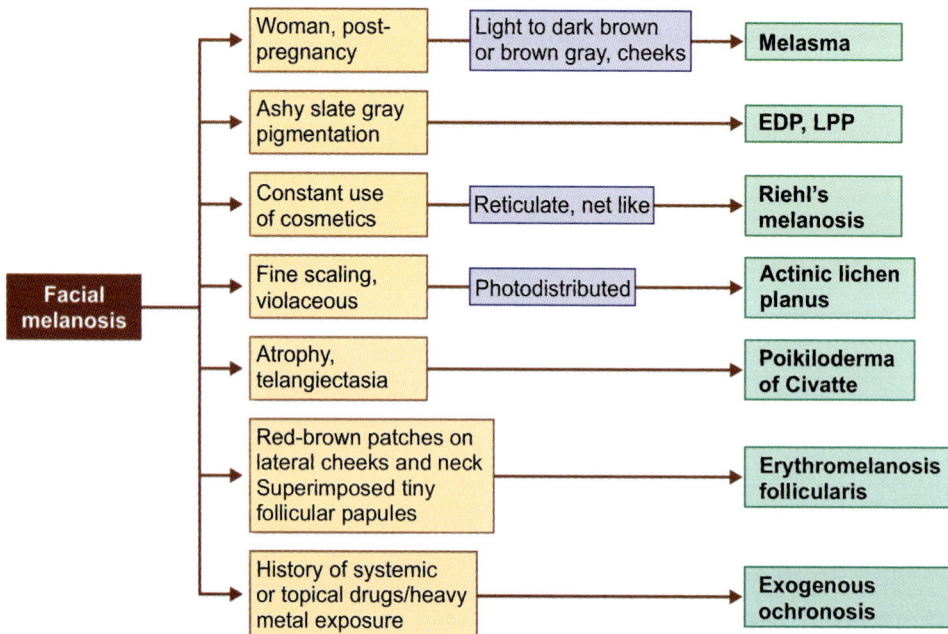

Fig. 4.1: Clinical approach to facial melanosis (EDP: Erythema dyschromicum perstans, LPP: Lichen planus pigmentosus)

1. COMMON DISORDERS

MELASMA

Introduction

Melasma is a very common acquired disorder of skin pigmentation characterized by presence of symmetrical light to dark brown pigmentation on the face affecting the malar area, cheeks, chin or forehead. Melasma is derived from the Greek word 'melas' which means 'black' and it is also referred to as 'chloasma' meaning 'the mask of pregnancy'.

Epidemiology

Melasma is a very common disorder and affects a sizeable percentage of the world population. It is much more common in females as compared to males and affects people with Fitzpatrick skin type III to V predominantly. The prevalence of this disease has been found to be about 8% in Hispanic females. In southeast Asia, the incidence has been reported to be in the range of 30–40%.

Melasma is a disease of reproductive age group and it is especially common in pregnant and lactating females. There is a premenstrual flare of the disease noticed by some females. In 41% of females, the onset of melasma is after pregnancy but before menopause while in the rest, the disease usually starts before pregnancy or marriage.

Melasma is seen in males as well and in southeast Asia, the ratio of males to females affected by melasma is about 1:2.

Etiopathogenesis

The exact etiopathogenesis of melasma is not known. It is believed that following exposure to an inducing or precipitating agent, there is increased production of melanin by hyperfunctional melanocytes in the affected skin. The most important of all precipitating agents is UV radiation and this is proved by the fading of melasma in winter months as well as the distribution of melasma lesions.

Other known precipitating and aggravating agents include oral contraceptive pills, pregnancy, emotional stress, autoimmune thyroid disease and drugs like phenytoin and other phototoxic drugs. Melasma is known to start or aggravate in pregnancy and postpartum period in females. Some mild hormonal imbalances have been reported in both females as well as males with melasma but the exact significance of these hormonal disturbances is not known.

Clinical Features

Melasma is characterized by the presence of light to dark brown macular pigmentation with irregular borders on the face. The pigmentation is distributed symmetrically on both sides of the face and may involve the malar area, cheeks, chin, upper lip and forehead in varying intensity.

On the basis of the pattern of involvement, melasma is divided into three main morphological types:

a. Centrofacial type—the most common form in which the forehead, cheeks, nose, upper lip and chin are involved.
b. Malar type—which involves the malar area and nose predominantly (Fig. 4.2a to c).
c. Mandibular type—which typically involves the jawline of the face (Fig. 4.2b).

The extent or severity of pigmentation in melasma varies from light brown to very dark brown or even brown-gray. More severe the pigmentation more difficult it is to treat the disease.

Melasma has also been divided on the basis of the depth or location of pigmentation into three types:

a. Epidermal—wherein the pigmentation is limited to the epidermis only (Fig. 4.2d);

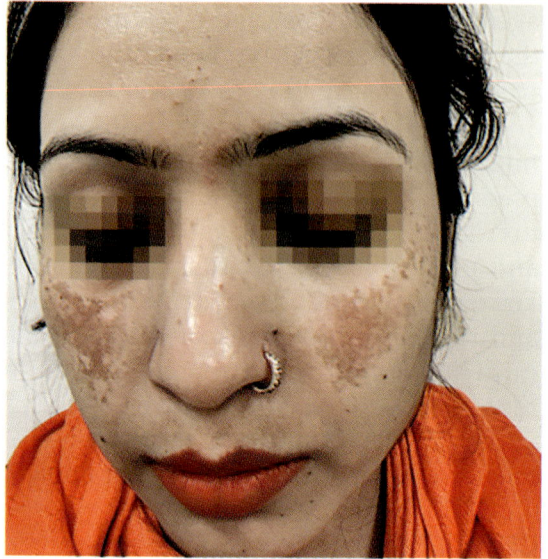

Fig. 4.2a: A young female with melasma involving the malar area. The lesions started in pregnancy

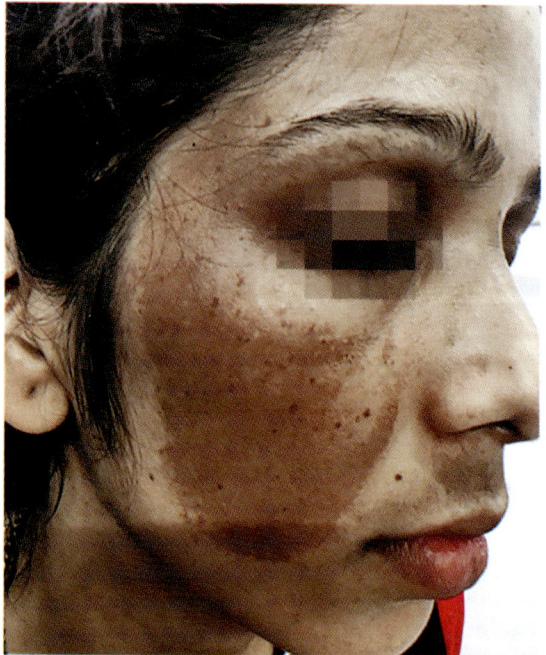

Fig. 4.2b: A 35-year-old female with malar and mandibular melasma. Also note the presence of freckles on cheeks

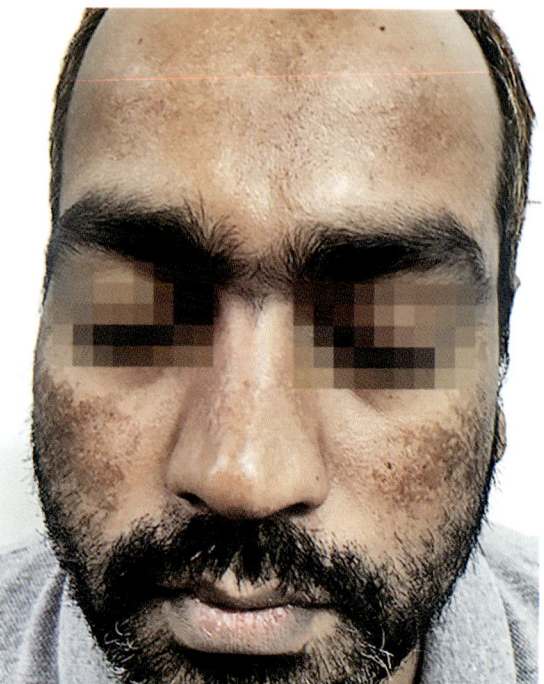

Fig. 4.2c: Malar melasma in a 35-year-old male. Melasma is rare in men. Unlike females, hormones play little role in pathogenesis. UV light and mustard oil are important causative factors in male melasma

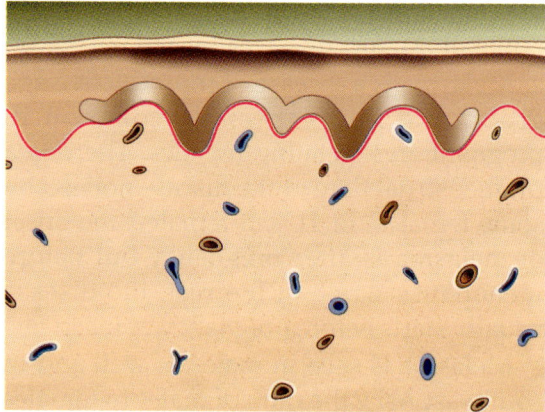

Fig. 4.2d: A case of melasma (epidermal) with increased melanin pigmentation in the basal layer

b. Mixed—wherein the epidermis as well as dermis are involved; and lastly

c. Dermal—where the pigmentation is limited to dermis only.

Theoretically, while epidermal melasma is accentuated under Wood's lamp, dermal pigmentation remains unchanged. This classification is, however, not favored now and people have questioned the presence of a pure dermal melasma.

Differential Diagnosis

Melasma needs to be differentiated from many other disorders that can cause facial pigmentation. These disorders and the differentiating points from melasma are given in Table 4.1.

Treatment

Treatment of a patient of melasma is done on multiple fronts.
1. General advice
2. Topical/systemic medications
3. Aesthetic procedures, if needed.

General Advice

The most important advice that needs to be passed onto a patient of melasma is diligent sun protection. This means the regular use of a broad-spectrum sunscreen with high UVA protection ability, use of hats or umbrellas and avoidance of habitual sun exposure as far as possible.

In addition, any known aggravating factors need to be taken care of like avoiding estrogen-containing oral contraceptives, avoiding other phototoxic drugs or treatment of any autoimmune thyroid disease.

Sunscreens form a very important constituent of melasma management and they should be applied regularly and liberally on the face both during summers as well as winters. Ideally, the sunscreen should provide a good protection against UVA light and should be cosmetically appealing to the patients. Sunscreens need to be applied twice or thrice daily and repeated after bathing or swimming.

Table 4.1: Differential diagnosis of melasma	
Disease	*Differentiating points*
1. Lichen planus pigmentosus (LPP)	1. Begins in temples and then involves the sides of the face and neck 2. Grayish black pigmentation
2. Riehl's melanosis	1. Grayish brown pigmentation usually involving the sides of the face and even neck or forehead. 2. Pigmentation may be reticulate in nature 3. Due to cosmetic use
3. Exogenous ochronosis	1. History of prolonged application of hydroquinone 2. History of aggravation of pigmentation after hydroquinone application 3. Micropapules or even pigmented papules may be present 4. Characteristic histology 5. Fine scaling over the pigmented lesions
4. Actinic lichen planus	1. Discrete pigmented macules 2. Halo of depigmentation
5. Poikiloderma of Civatte	1. Involvement of anterior neck 2. Atrophy and telangiectasia
6. Pigmented photocontact dermatitis	1. Areas of sides of forehead and cheeks commonly involved. 2. History of application of oils or perfumed substances on face or scalp. 3. Presence of inflammatory signs especially in early stages

Drug Therapy

Topical drug therapy is the mainstay of treatment of melasma. Majority of drugs used for melasma basically target the melanin production by inhibiting the rate limiting enzyme tyrosinase. These drugs and their main mechanism of action are given in Table 4.2.

Hydroquinone is the most extensively used topical drug in melasma. It acts by inhibiting the enzyme tyrosinase leading to inhibition of melanin synthesis. Scientific studies have documented the efficacy and safety of this molecule in pigmentary disorders including melasma. The only concern is the development of exogenous ochronosis on long-term use of this drug especially when used in higher concentrations. In addition, hydroquinone can also lead to irritant and allergic contact dermatitis and post-inflammatory hyperpigmentation.

Retinoids are the other class of drugs used commonly in the treatment of melasma. Retinoids can be used as monotherapy in melasma but more commonly they are used in combination with hydroquinone and topical steroids. In fact, one of the most commonly used treatment option in melasma is a combination of hydroquinone, tretinoin and a mild topical steroid like hydrocortisone or flucinolone. The credit of developing this combination goes to Kligman who first described the formula. This original Kligman's formula has been modified over years and the most common combination used nowadays contains hydroquinone 2%, tretinoin 0.025% and flucinolone acetonide 0.1%.

In India, there are combinations of hydroquinone, tretinoin and mometasone available which are used rampantly by general practitioners. These combinations are, however, associated with a lot of adverse effects like skin atrophy, telangiectasia, acne and hypertrichosis and should not be prescribed ideally. And even if they are prescribed, they should be used for the minimum possible duration of less than 2–3 weeks (Majid).

Various agents used for the treatment of hyperpigmentation are described in Chapter 7.

Aesthetic Procedures

Patients who do not respond to topical agents or who want a more rapid response are managed by certain aesthetic procedures which usually act in combination with topical agents. These procedures include peels, lasers and miscellaneous procedures.

Peeling or chemexfoliation constitutes the most commonly used procedure in melasma. Among peeling agents, glycolic acid is not only the most commonly used but probably the most efficacious as well. Other peeling agents used in melasma are salicylic acid, mandelic acid, lactic acid and also tretinoin (Hurley).

Peels, however, have to be used with caution as they can lead to post-inflammatory hyperpigmentation especially in colored or dark skin. Measures that can minimize the chances of this adverse effect are pre-peel priming of the skin with hydroquinone, judicious selection and use of

Table 4.2: Topical agents used in melasma	
Topical agent	Mechanism of action
Hydroquinone	Tyrosinase inhibitor Increased melanosome destruction
Arbutin	Tyrosinase inhibitor Inhibition of melanosome maturation
Licorice extract	Tyrosinase inhibitor
Rucinol	Tyrosinase inhibitor
Azelaic acid	Tyrosinase inhibitor
Retinoids	Increased melanocyte turnover Reduction in melanosome transfer
Ascorbic acid	Interaction with copper
Kojic acid	Interaction with copper

peeling agents, doing a test-peel before the procedure and post-peel sun avoidance.

In addition to peels, other less commonly used procedures in melasma are microdermabrasion and lasers. However, all these procedures have their own limitations and can lead to aggravation of disease in some cases. As of now, these procedures are not recommended in treatment of melasma.

Whatever the treatment chosen, it needs to be understood that melasma is associated with relapse whenever the treatment is stopped. This calls for the use of safer treatment options without any propensity to cause adverse effects and maintenance treatment regimens with absolutely safe drugs to prevent relapses.

Bibliography

1. Ennes SBP, Paschoalick RC, Mota de Avelar Alchorne M. A double-blind, comparative, placebo-controlled study of the efficacy and tolerability of 4% hydroquinone as a depigmenting agent in melasma. J Dermatol Treat 2000; 11:173–9.

2. Gilchrest BA, Fitzpatrick TB, Anderson RR, Parrish JA. Localization of melanin pigmentation in the skin with Wood's lamp. Br J Dermatol 1977;96: 245–8.

3. Grimes PE. Melasma: Etiologic and therapeutic considerations. Arch Dermatol 1995;131:1453–7.

4. Gupta AK, Gover MD, Nouri K, Taylor S. The treatment of melasma: A review of clinical trials. J Am Acad Dermatol 2006;55:1048–69.

5. Hurley ME, Guevara IL, Gonzales RM, Pandya AG. Efficacy of glycolic acid peels in the treatment of melasma. Arch Dermatol 2002;138:1578–82.

6. Jimbow K, Obata H, Pathak M, Fitzpatrick TB. Mechanism of depig-mentation by hydroquinone. J Invest Dermatol 1974;62:436–49.

7. Kramer K, Lopez A, Stefanato C, Phillips TJ. Exogenous ochronosis. J Am Acad Dermatol 2000; 42:869–71.

8. Lakhdar H, Zouhair K, Khadir K, Essari A, Richard A, Seite S, et al. Evaluation of the effectiveness of broad-spectrum sunscreen in the prevention of chloasma in pregnant women. J Eur Acad Dermatol Venereol 2007;21:738–42.

9. Majid I. Mometasone based triple combination therapy in melasma: Is it really safe? Indian J Dermatol 2010;55:359–62.

10. Ortonne JP, Arellano I, Berneburg M, Cestari T, Chan H, Grimes P, et al. A global survey of the role of ultraviolet radiation and hormonal influences in the development of melasma. J Eur Acad Dermatol Venereol 2009;23:1254–62.

11. Perez M, Sanchez JL, Aguilo F. Endocrinologic profile of patients with idiopathic melasma. J Invest Dermatol1983;81:543–5.

12. Resnik S. Melasma induced by oral contraceptive drugs. JAMA 1967;199:601–5.

13. Sanchez NP, Pathak MA, Sato S. Melasma: A clinical, light micro-scopic, ultrastructural, and immunofluorescence study. J Am Acad Dermatol 1981;4:698–709.

14. Sheth VM, Pandya AG. Melasma: A comprehensive update Part II. J Am Acad Dermatol 2011;65: 699–714.

15. Sivayathorn A. Melasma in Orientals. Clin Drug Invest 1995; 10:34–40.

16. Tayior SC, Torok H, Jones T, Lowe N, Rich P, Tschen E, et al. Efficacy and safety of a new triple-combination agent for the treatment of facial melasma. Cutis 2003;72:67–72.

17. Werlinger KD, Guevara IL, Gonzalez CM, Rincon ET, Caetano R, Haley RW, et al. Prevalence of self-diagnosed melasma among pre-menopausal Latino women in Dallas and Forth Worth, Tex. Arch Dermatol 2007; 143:424–5.

FRECKLES (EPHELIDES) AND LENTIGINES

Clinical Features

Freckles are small round/oval or irregular shaped pigmented spots, generally reddish to pale brown in color, which commonly appear on the exposed body parts, namely face, neck, chest and arms, of fair phototype individuals, particularly in those with red hair. They are relatively uniform in distribution, size and color. The spots are mostly less than 3 mm and have poorly defined lateral margins (Fig. 4.3a). Freckles appear during the childhood years and partially disappear with age. They become darker in the summer months and fade during the

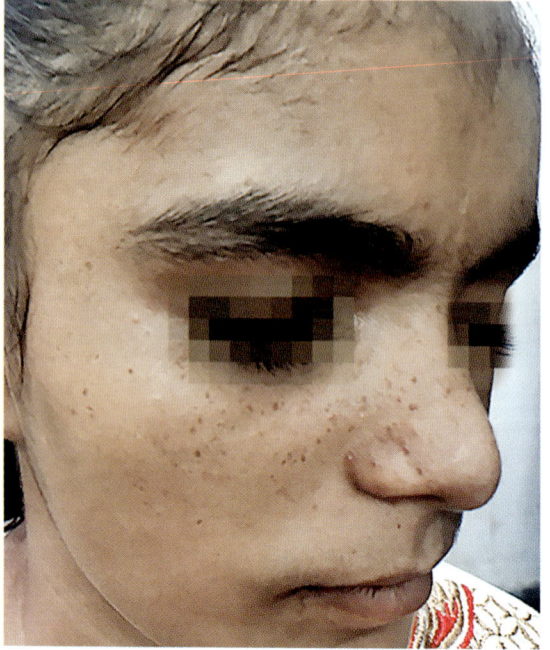

Fig. 4.3a: Freckles

ageing and chronic sun exposure. These pigmented spots have well-defined smooth or irregular borders and vary in color from light to dark brown (darker than freckles). The lighter spots appear homogenous in color, while the larger ones appear mottled. The size is also variable and ranges from a few millimetres to several centimetres (larger than freckles). Also, solar lentigines, unlike freckles, are non-uniformly distributed over the sun-exposed sites, often on a background of other signs of photoaging. Most common sites affected are the dorsa of hands and forearms, face, upper chest and back. In contrast to freckles, solar lentigines persist indefinitely and show no seasonal variation. The underlying pathology is a UV exposure induced proliferation of basal melanocytes and a subsequent increase in their melanization.

The term 'lentiginosis' is used when lentigines are present in large numbers or when they occur in a distinctive distribution. Lentiginosis may be a component of various genetic syndromes.

PUVA lentigines and ink spot lentigo are the other types of lentigines, which develop after PUVA therapy and intense sun exposure, respectively. Lentigo simplex or simple lentigo are smaller spots (generally <5 mm), which can appear as multiple lesions, involving both the exposed and unexposed parts, particularly in those with fair skin and red hair. Multiple simple lentigines may occur as an isolated phenomenon or in association with various syndromes involving internal organs as well.

Rarely, in syndromes, lentigines may involve the mucosa (Fig. 4.3b and c).

The clinical significance, of both freckles and lentigines, lies in the fact that they are both markers of excessive sun exposure and some risk of skin cancer.

winters. The underlying mechanism is an increase in local melanin production, following UV exposure, in genetically predisposed individuals.

Freckling without associated abnormalities is transmitted in an autososmal dominant fashion.

Extensive freckling may also occur as a part of the photosensitive genodermatosis—xeroderma pigmentosum. Axillary and inguinal freckling is one of the diagnostic criteria of neurofibromatosis type 1 syndrome. However, it is believed that these 'freckles' are actually small cafe au' lait macules.

Solar lentigines are markers of photoaging, and thus increase in number and prevalence with age. They are not associated with any particular skin type or hair color. The different names used for solar lentigines, i.e. sun-induced freckles, sunburn freckles, freckles in adulthood, lentigo senilis, age spot and actinic lentigines, also reflect their well-established link with

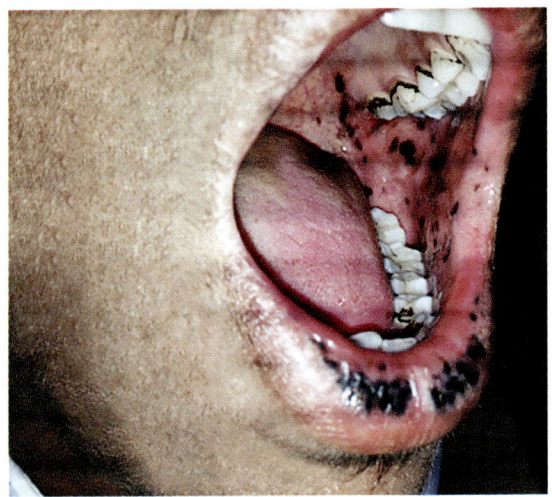

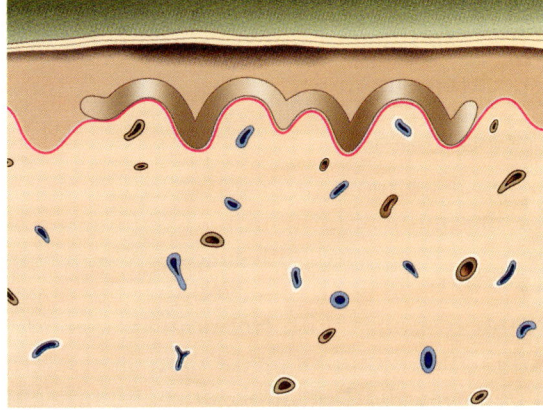

Fig. 4.3d: Increased pigmentation in the basal layer without increase in melanocytes

Fig. 4.3b: Mucosal lentigines in a young male. Evaluation revealed polyps in small intestine (Peutz-Jeghers syndrome)

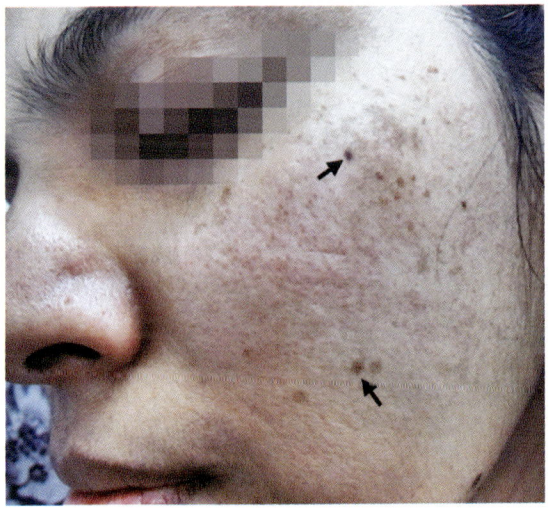

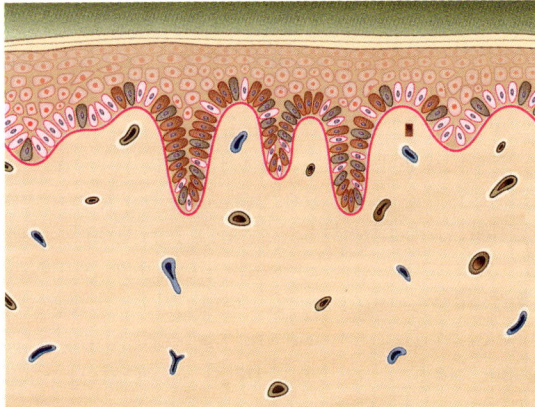

Fig. 4.3e: Increased basal layer pigmentation due to increase in both melnocytes and melanin. Note that the rete-ridges are elongated

Investigations

No investigations need to be carried out in a simple case of freckles or lentigines, unless an associated genetic disorder is suspected.

Treatment

General Advice

Fig. 4.3c: Lentigines in a female patient. Note the well-defined margins. The lesions did not have a seasonal variation

Diagnosis

The diagnosis of freckles and lentigines is based on their clinical appearance only. Histopathology reveals no discernible abnormality (except an increase in quantity of melanin) in a freckle, while a lentigo would show a linear increase in the number of melanocytes at the epidermal–dermal junction (Fig. 4.3d and e).

Most important component in the management of freckles and lentigines is sun protection. The patient needs to be sensitized to this aspect of treatment to achieve any significant clinical benefit. Various cosmetically acceptable and even tinted sunscreens are now available. Use of protective gear is also essential in addition to the use of broad-spectrum sunscreens.

Topical Therapy

Topical tretinoin (0.05–0.1%), either alone, or in combination with hydroquinone (2–4%) has been used with success. Kligman et al. and Rafal et al. observed that the maximum response with tretinoin is achieved when the amount of medication used is to a point just short of intolerance. Significant improvement may take a long time to develop with tretinoin alone, and the patient needs to be counselled well regarding the expected adverse effects. On the up side though, improvement in other signs of photoaging is also observed with the prolonged use of tretinoin.

Use in combination with hydroquinone hastens the onset of action. The triple combination (modified) Kligman's formula is also a commonly prescribed agent for freckles and solar lentigines. However, the prolonged use of hydroquinone and steroids should be discouraged, as it has been associated with various local adverse effects. Exogenous ochronosis is a particularly distressing and largely irreversible adverse effect seen with long-term unsupervised use of hydroqui-none. It is characterized by bluish brown pigmentation with interspersed "confetti like" hypopigmented macules. The effects of prolonged steroid use are well known and include atrophy, telangiectasias and loss of pigment.

Chemical Peel

Chemical peels, either spot or full face, are to be performed by a trained dermatologist only. Glycolic acid is the most commonly used agent in this regard. Low concentration (<35%) trichloracetic acid (TCA) and 88% phenol can be applied over the freckles, but often leave behind bothersome hypo-/depigmentation.

Cosmetic Therapy

Destructive modalities, like cryotherapy, are also recommended for lentigines. However, this may lead to significant dyspigmentation in dark-skinned individuals.

Q-switched (Qs) ruby, alexandrite and Nd:YAG lasers are recognised to be effective in the treatment of freckles and lentigines. Post-inflammatory hyperpigmentation (PIH) is an important side effect which occurs in about 10–25% of cases in Asians. Ho et al. used long pulsed (LP) lasers to circumvent this problem and reported good

Table 4.3: Overview of the management of freckles/lentigines			
	Medical management	*Cosmetic intervention*	*Laser/surgery*
Topical	Sunscreens (most essential) Topical retinoids Hydroquinone Modified Kligman formula Mequinol Arbutin Deoxyarbutin Adapalene Azelaic acid Ascorbic acid	**Chemical peels** (Glycolic acid and tretinoin) **Spot peel**	**Cryotherapy** **Lasers** Qs red and infrared lasers Fractional CO_2 resurfacing
Level of care	**Primary**	**Tertiary** Refer to dermatologist	**Tertiary** Refer to dermatologist

response, without PIH, with the use of 595 nm long pulsed dye laser (LPDL) and 532 nm LP potassium-titanyl-phosphate (KTP) laser, in Chinese patients. No significant improvement was found after LP alexandrite laser. Also, PIH risk was 20% after LP alexandrite treatment and 10% with Qs Nd:YAG. The use of fractional carbon dioxide laser has also been associated with a good overall outcome.

An overview of the management is given in Table 4.3.

Bibliography

1. Bastiaens M, Hoefnagel J, Westendorp R, et al. Solar lentigines are strongly related to sun exposure in contrast to ephelides. Pigment Cell Res 2004; 17(3):225–9.

2. Chan HH, Fung WKK, Ying SY, et al. An in vivo trial comparing the use of different types of 532-nm Nd:YAG lasers in the treatment of facial lentigines in oriental patients. Derm Surg 2000;26: 743–9.

3. El Zawahry B, Zaki N, Hafez V, et al. Efficacy and safety of fractional carbon dioxide laser for treatment of unwanted facial freckles in phototypes II-IV: A pilot study. Lasers Med Sci 2014 Nov; 29:1937–42.

4. Ezzedine K, Mauger E, Latreille J, et al. Freckles and solar lentigines have different risk factors in Caucasian women. J Eur Acad Dermatol Venereol 2013; 27(3):e345–56.

5. Ho SG, Chan NP, Yeung CK, et al. A retrospective analysis of the management of freckles and lentigines using four different pigment lasers on Asian skin. J Cosmet Laser Ther 2012; 14(2):74–80.

6. Ho SG, Chan NP, Yeung CK, et al. A retrospective analysis of the management of freckles and lentigines using fourdifferent pigment lasers on Asian skin. Cosmet Laser Ther 2012;14:74–80.

7. Kligman AM. Guidelines for the use of topical tretinoin (Retin-A) for photoaged skin. J Am Acad Dermatol 1989; 21 (3 Pt 2):650–4.

8. Liu WC, Tey HL, Lee JS, et al. Exogenous ochronosis in a Chinese patient: Use of dermoscopy aids early diagnosis and selection of biopsy site. Singapore Med J 2014; 55(1):e1–3.

9. Murphy MJ, Huang MY. Q-switched ruby laser treatment of benign pigmented lesions in Chinese skin. Am Acad Med Singapore 1994;23:60–66.

10. Newton Bishop JA. Lentigos, melanocytic nevi and melanoma. In Burns T, Breathnach S, Cox N, Griffiths C eds. Rook's textbook of Dermatology, 8th ed., UK: Wiley-Blackwell 2010: 54.10–54.56.

11. Ortonne JP1, Pandya AG, Lui H, et al. Treatment of solar lentigines. J Am Acad Dermatol 2006; 54(5 Suppl 2):S262–71.

12. Rabinovitz HS, Barnhill RL. Benign Melanocytic neoplasms. In Bolognia JL, Jorizzo JL, Schaffer JV eds. Dermatology, 3rd edition, Elsevier Saunders 2012:1857–85.

13. Rafal ES, Griffiths CE, Ditre CM, et al. Topical tretinoin (retinoic acid) treatment for liver spots associated with photodamage. N Engl J Med 1992; 326(6):368–74.

14. Wang CC, Sue YM, Yang CH, et al. A comparison of Q-switched alexandrite laser and intense pulsed light for the treatment of freckles and lentigines in Asian persons: A randomised, physician-blinded, split-face comparative trial. J Am Acad Dermatol 2006; 54:804–10.

DERMATOSIS PAPULOSA NIGRA (DPN) AND SEBORRHEIC KERATOSIS

DPN is a common finding in African-American, Afro-Caribbean and sub-Saharan black patients. It is considered a variant of seborrheic keratoses, with an earlier age of onset in many cases.

These appear as flattened dark brown or black papules around 1–5 mm in diameter mainly over the malar area of face and forehead (Fig. 4.4a and b). DPN are asymptomatic and can be removed with diathermy or cautery, if the patient desires.

MATURATIONAL HYPERPIGMENTATION (MH)

This condition was first described by Dr A. Melvin Alexander, who first noticed what he calls "maturational hyperpigmentation"—a mysterious disorder that predominantly affects blacks—when his brother, an otolaryngologist, developed it.

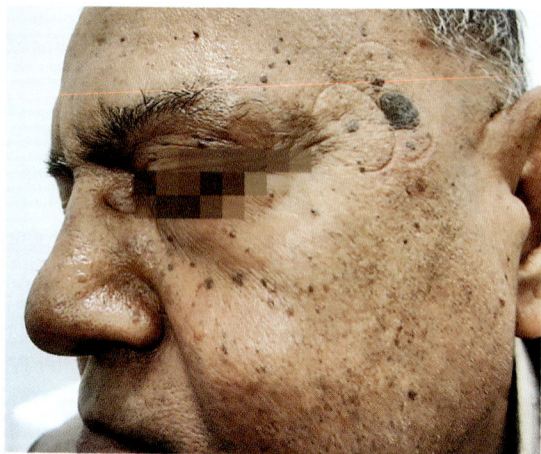

Fig. 4.4a: DPN: Multiple dark brown papules over the forehead and malar area of face in an elderly male. Also note the larger lesion in left temporal region that is suggestive of seborrheic keratosis

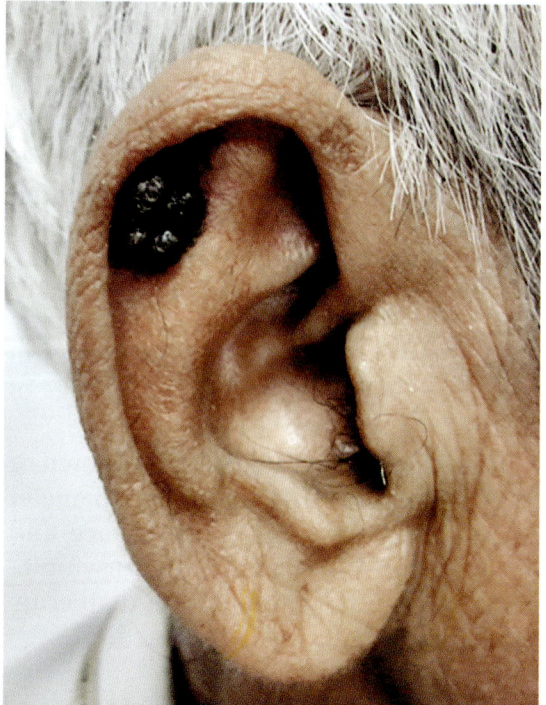

Fig. 4.4b: Multiple hyperkeratotic hyperpigmented papules coalescing to form a plaque on the ear in an elderly male. The lesions are classical of seborrheic keratoses

Maturational hyperpigmentation (MH) is a common entity seen among African-Americans and other people of color who have various allergies and a diabetic diathesis. It is specially common in India and is possibly related to insulin resistance.

Clinical Features

Clinically, MH appears on the cheeks, especially the malar eminences, forehead and face as a diffuse melasma-like hyperpigmentation (Figs 4.5 and 4.6). However, unlike melasma, it has ill-defined borders that fade into the person's normal skin color. Melasma usually has a medium brown color, whereas MH has a dark brown to black color. It may be unilateral or bilateral. In Indians, the skin is visibly thickened and the morphology is akin to acanthosis nigricans. It usually occurs in the 4th–5th decade of life.

The possible causes include friction, DM, hyperglycemia and insulin resistance. Interestingly of the seven patients, described initially, where melanocyte-stimulating hormone (MSH) was measured, six (86%) showed low levels of this hormone, which is surprising considering the clinical hyperpigmentation and the melanocyte proliferation seen in the biopsies. MH may be a "new" cutaneous marker for diabetes or prediabetes.

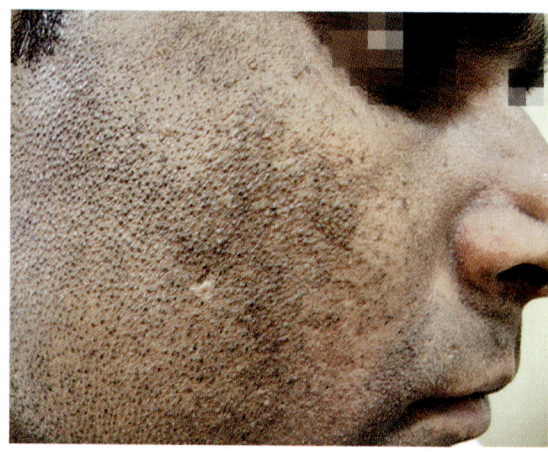

Fig. 4.5: Maturational hyperpigmentation (face)

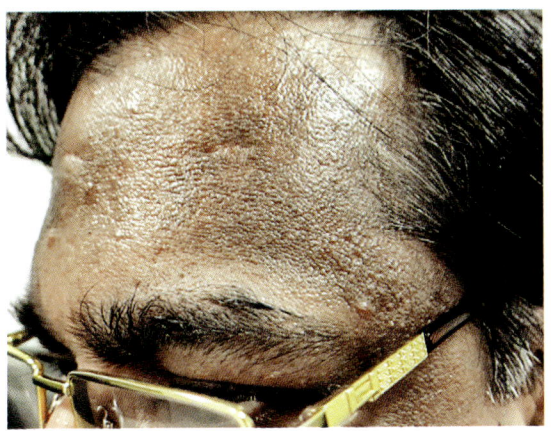

Fig. 4.6a: Maturational hyperpigmentation (forehead)

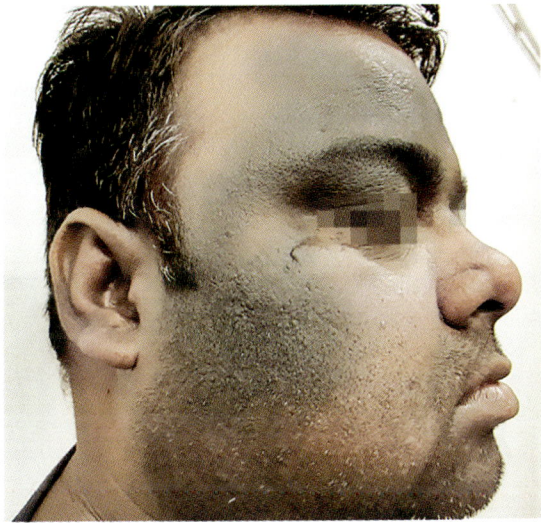

Fig. 4.6b: Facial acanthosis nigricans in a young male with metabolic syndrome. Maturational hyperpigmentation and facial AN are considered synonymous by many authors though there are subtle differences between the two entities

Skin biopsy reveals melanocyte proliferation, papillomatous epidermal proliferation with minimal or absent dermal inflammation.

Investigations

1. Insulin levels and HOMA-IR (homeostatic model-assessment estimated insulin resistance) calculation
2. Blood sugar levels
3. Thyroid function test

Treatment

Therapy has not been consistently successful using hydroquinones, topical retinoids, and/or mild corticosteroids or microdermabrasion. Lasers have also been tried but with disappointing results.

Bibliography

Pigmentation Disorders. In. Sardana K, Garg VK, Mahajan S, eds. Diagnosis and Management of Skin Diseases: An Evidence Based Approach, Wolters Kluwer, LWW 2012, 1st edition.

PERIORBITAL HYPERMELANOSIS (PIGMENTATION)

Periorbital hyperpigmentation, often colloquially referred to as dark circles, is defined as bilateral, homogeneous hyperchromic macules and patches primarily involving the upper and lower eyelids but also sometimes extending towards the eyebrows, malar regions, and lateral nasal root. An Indian study showed that it is most prevalent in the age group of 16 to 25 years and is more common in women

There are various causes including genetics, fatigue, stress, emotional lability, exhaustion of the periorbital muscles and aging. Lifestyle factors associated with periorbital hyperpigmentation may include alcohol overuse, smoking, and excessive drinking (Table 4.4). In an Indian study, it was found that POH was an extension of the pigmentary demarcation line (described below) over the face in 92% of patients.

Clinical Features

The clinical presentation of periorbital hyperpigmentation is related to its pathogenesis:

1. Periorbital hyperpigmentation secondary to excessive epidermal melanin may appear brown in color (Fig. 4.7a to c).
2. Pigmentation secondary to excessive dermal melanin may appear blue-gray in color.

Table 4.4: Etiology of periorbital hyperpigmentation

Most common	Fatigue/stress Hereditary factors Aging/photodamage Lifestyle factors (alcohol, smoking, caffeine)
Dermatological causes	Postinflammatory Atopy Eye strain Hormonal Medications (oral contraceptives, antipsychotics, chemotherapeutics, etc.)
Systemic causes	Hepatic/renal disease Thyroid disease Addison disease Carcinoma Ecchymoses Vitamin K deficiency Hereditary blood disorder

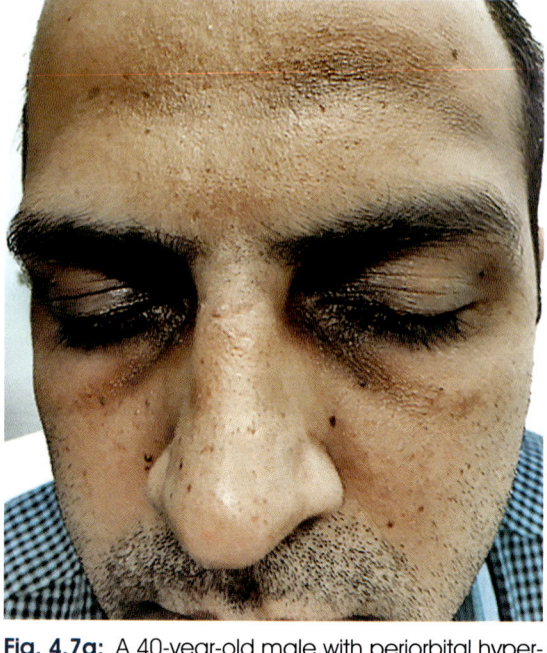

Fig. 4.7a: A 40-year-old male with periorbital hypermelanosis

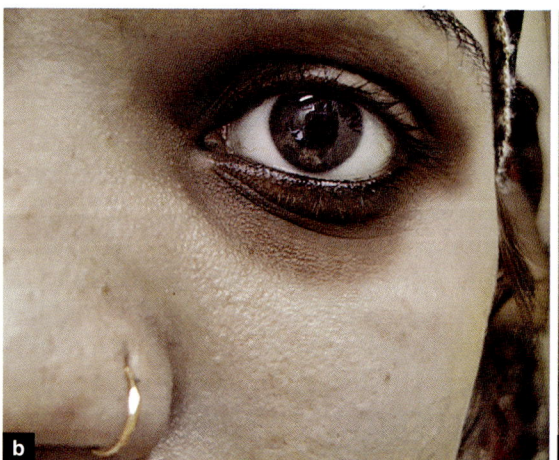

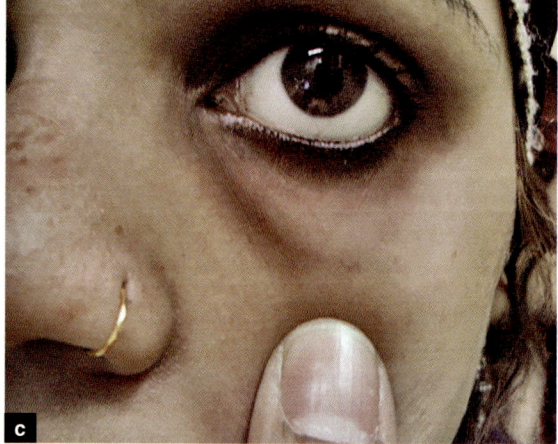

Fig. 4.7b and c: (b) Periorbital pigmentation which approximates the shape of the inferior orbital margin; (c) Manual stretching of the lower eyelid leads to no obvious change of the pigments

3. Periorbital hyperpigmentation related to hypervascularity often has a violaceous or bluish color owing to visibility of the dermal capillary network. The violaceous hue accentuates on manual stretching of lower eyelid. Periorbital hyperpigmentation owing to periorbital edema is often characterized by variability, a purplish hue, and is often worse in the morning or after a salty meal.

4. Pseudoherniation of the periorbital fat and skin laxity can result in the creation of dark shadows. Facial movements may cause repositioning of the muscles and

skin, thus altering the pattern of light on the face and emphasizing the appearance of hyperpigmentation.

Diagnosis

POH is diagnosed mainly by clinical examination. True pigmentation should be differentiated from shadowing effect. This can be done by manual stretching of the skin of lower eyelid. True pigmentation remains the same whereas shadowing due to tear trough improves or resolves completely.

Treatment

Prognosis depends on identification and management of the primary causes of hyperpigmentation. Unfortunately, even with a thorough understanding of etiologic factors, periorbital hyperpigmentation may remain recalcitrant to therapeutic intervention. Proper management of patient expectations, therefore, is paramount.

The treatment depends on the cause (Fig. 4.7d):

1. If the cause is due to pigmentation in the skin, various topical preparations may work. This includes HQ, azelaic acid, kojic acid, licorice, arbutin, glycolic acid, vitamin C. Steroids should be

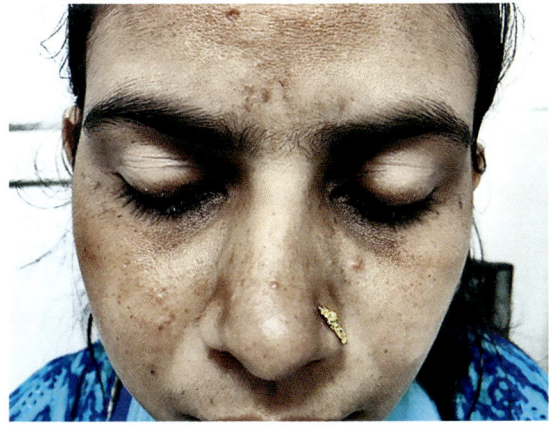

Fig. 4.7d: A female with periorbital hypermelanosis with lightening of pigmentation on chemical peels containing arginine, lactic acid and kojic acid

avoided. Though chemical peels have been tried, they should be used with caution. Glycolic acid 20%, lactic acid 15%, and arginine are the agents used for chemical peels in periorbital region. It should be noted that when periorbital hyperpigmentation is caused primarily by hypervascularity, chemical peels are contraindicated because they may worsen the clinical appearance.

2. If the cause is due to dermal melanin, lasers may be tried. Q-switched ruby laser (694 nm), Q-switched alexandrite laser, and Nd:YAG (1064 nm) laser have been tried for treating dark circles.

3. If the cause is due to "laxity of skin", Botox and surgical options are advised. Botulinum toxin type A may help to lessen the appearance of periorbital hyperpigmentation in cases where active musculature alters the pattern of light on the face and emphasizes dark shadows. Restylane (hyaluronic acid) is the most popular filler for ethnic skin and may be used to fill periorbital hollows and to restore volume, thus decreasing shadowing.

   Thin eyelid skin can be treated with autologous fat transplantation. Platelet-rich plasma therapy has been tried in patients with tear trough deformities and wrinkles with good results.

   Blepharoplasty, either alone or in conjunction with other procedures, may be useful in eliminating periorbital hyperpigmentation caused by shadows cast by fat deposits and skin laxity. Transconjunctival blepharoplasty, coupled with phenol peels, has been reported to be effective in darker skin types.

4. *Cosmeceuticals*: Although response may be modest, over-the-counter cosmetics can improve the appearance

Table 4.5: Overview of the treatment of infraorbital pigmentation

	Medical management	*Cosmetic intervention*	*Laser/surgery*
Topical	Hydroquinone 2/4% Azelaic acid Kojic acid Vitamin C Vitamin K Alpha arbutin Niacinamide Glycolic acid Sunscreen	Chemical peeling Dermal fillers Botox	Lasers Surgical intervention (blepharoplasty)
Systemic	—		
Level of care	**Primary**	**Tertiary** Refer to dermatologist	**Tertiary** Refer to dermatologist

of periorbital hyperpigmentation temporarily by helping to restore moisture and tone. A topical product containing growth factors obtained from cultured human foreskin fibroblasts, TNS (Skin Medica Co.), may help to diminish periorbital pigmentation. Topical preparations containing vitamin K may be of some benefit because of their effect on the clotting mechanism. There are also many highly effective cosmetic concealers that can more than adequately mask the appearance of periorbital hyperpigmentation.

5. *Sunscreens*: Broad spectrum sunscreens and UV-coated sunglasses may help in improvement of POH.

Traditional Indian Remedy

Some Indian remedies that can be used include turmeric (curcumurin) and ghee. The former is now a part of many topical agents for melasma. In fact scientific research on curcumurin has found it to help by molecular mechanisms. Other treatments recommended include flax seed and almond oil. An overview of the treatment is given below (Table 4.5).

Bibliography

1. Downie JB. Esthetic considerations for ethnic skin. Semin Cutan Med Surg 2006; 25:158.

2. Freitag FM, Cestari TF. What causes dark circles under the eyes. J Cosmet Dermatol 2007; 6:211.

3. Gendler EC. Treatment of periorbital hyperpigmentation. Aesthet Surg J 2005; 25:618.

4. Hosoya T, Nakata A, Yamasaki F, Abas F, Shaari K, Lajis NH, Morita H. Curcumin-like diarylpentanoid analogues as melanogenesis inhibitors. J Nat Med 2012 Jan;66(1):166–76.

5. Malakar S, Lahiri K, Banerjee U, et al. Periorbital melanosis is an extension of pigmentary demarcation line-F on face. Indian J Dermatol Venereol Leprol 2007; 73:323–325.

6. Maruri CA, Diaz LA. Dark circles around the eyes. Cutis 1969; 5:979.

7. Park SY, Jin ML, Kim YH, Kim Y, Lee SJ. Aromatic-turmerone inhibits -MSH and IBMX-induced melanogenesis by inactivating CREB and MITF signaling pathways. Arch Dermatol Res 2011 Dec; 303(10):737–44.

8. Sheth PB, Shah HA, Dave JN. Periorbital hypeprigmentation: a study of its prevalence, common causative factors and its association with personal habits and other disorders. Indian J Dermatol 2014; 59:151–157.

9. Tu CX, Lin, M, Lu SS, Qi XY, Zhang RX, Zhang YY. Curcumin inhibits melanogenesis in human melanocytes. Phytother Res 2012 Feb;26(2): 174–9.

PIGMENTARY DEMARCATION LINES

They are also known as Futcher's or Voigt's lines and are physiological, abrupt transitions from deeper pigmented skin to lighter pigmented skin. These are most notable in dark skin individuals.

Clinical Features

The dorsal skin surfaces are relatively hyper-pigmented compared to the ventral surfaces. In individuals with darkly pigmented skin, visible lines of demarcation between dorsal and ventral surfaces are more conspicuous, especially on the anterolateral portion of the upper arm (Fig. 4.8). These demarcation lines are bilateral, symmetric and present from infancy through adulthood. However, majority of these lines become apparent in

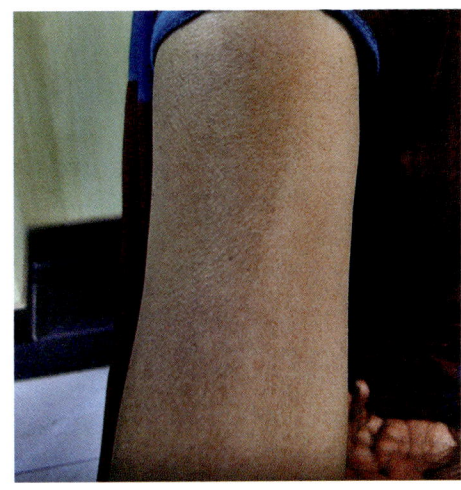

Fig. 4.8: PDL line type A. This is often treated with topical triple combination cream with little results

childhood. Additional lines are described below (Fig. 4.9).

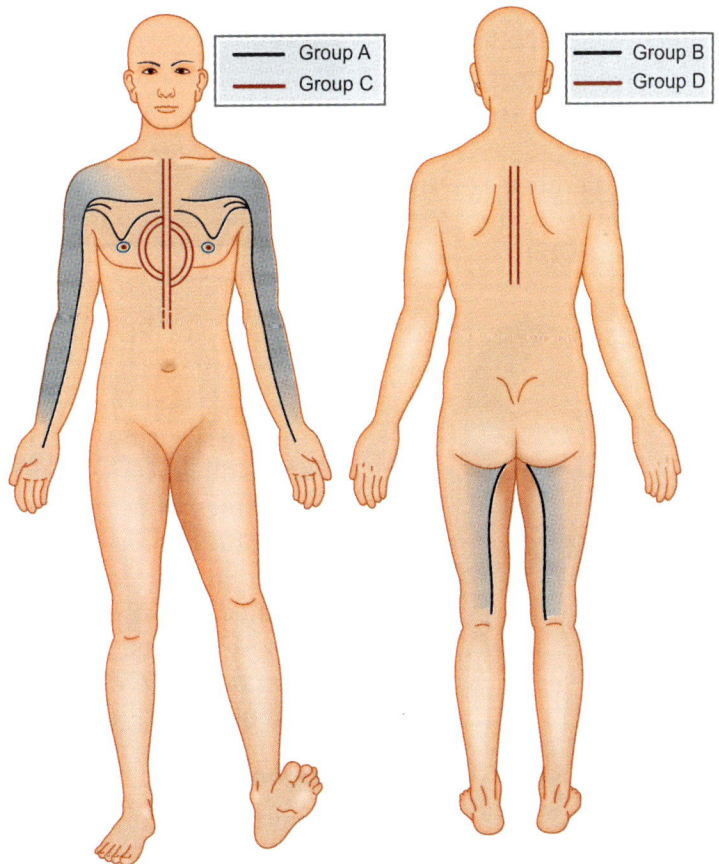

Fig. 4.9: A depiction of PDL on the body

a. On the lateral aspect of the upper arm extending over the pectoral area.

b. On the posteromedial portion of the lower limb.

c. Mediosternal line, a vertical hypopigmented line in the pre- and parasternal area.

d. On the posteromedial area of the spine, and

e. Bilateral hypopigmented streaks, bands or lanceolate areas over the chest in the zone between the mid-third of the clavicle and the periareolar skin.

On the face, three lines (Fig. 4.10) have been described and are relevant as they are frequently misdiagnosed and treated as melasma. Some of the lines specially type 'F' and 'G' actually has an infraorbital extension.

a. V-shaped hyperpigmented lines between the malar prominence and the temple.

b. W-shaped hyperpigmented lines between the malar prominence and the temple (Fig. 4.11).

c. Linear bands of hyperpigmentation from the angle of the mouth to the lateral aspects of the chin (Fig. 4.12).

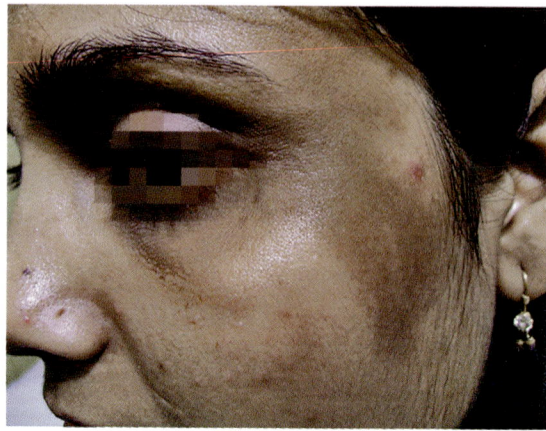

Fig. 4.11: A patient with a PDL line "G" on the face

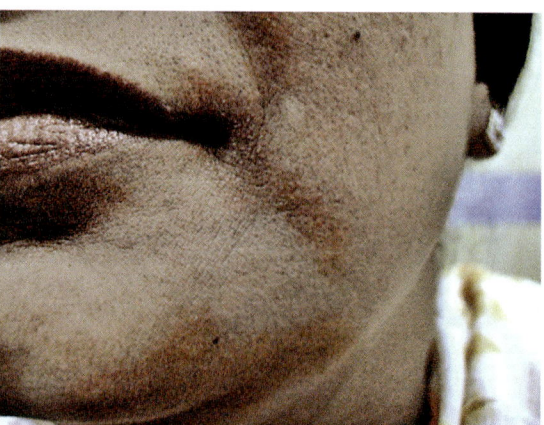

Fig. 4.12: PDL line "H" on the face

Etiology of PDL is unknown. Various theories have been postulated for this entity. Some authors proposed that PDL coincide with distribution of cutaneous nerves whereas others have hypothesized that they follow lines of Blaschko and is related to pigmentary mosaicism. PDL have been reported to occur in pregnancy and this may be related to neurogenic inflammation in this condition due to compression of S1 and S2 peripheral nerves of the spinal cord by the gravid uterus. It is exclusively group B PDL.

Diagnosis

Facial PDLs can often be misdiagnosed as melasma, post-inflammatory pigmentation, nevus of Ota or Ito, or melanocytic nevus.

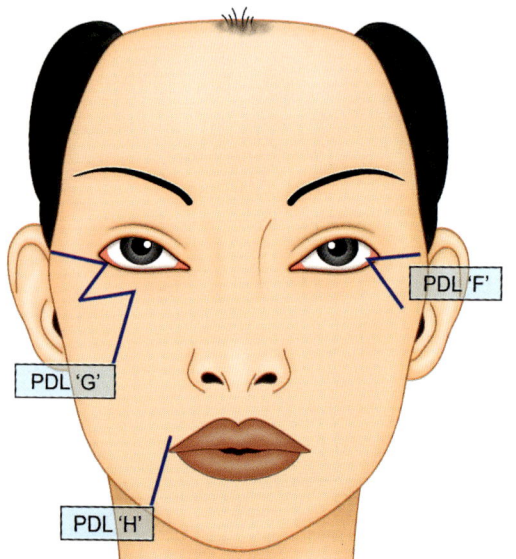

PDL 'F'

PDL 'G'

PDL 'H'

Fig. 4.10: A depiction of PDL on the face

Melasma occurs as a blotchy pigmentation over the malar areas just below the PDL F, and may involve other parts of the face like the nose, supraorbital areas or upper lips. Nevus of Ota has a bluish or greenish black color and a scleral component. PDL should also be differentiated from post-inflammatory hyperpigmentation (PIH). The latter will have prior history of skin lesions and ill-defined margins. A few authors believe that facial PDL and familial periorbital hyperpigmentation may represent the same entity.

Treatment

No therapy works and it is better to inform the patient accordingly instead of giving steroid based cream, triple combination creams that cause side effects or non-HQ based creams that are ineffective in this condition. Chemical peels (with glycolic acid) and Q-switched alexandrite laser have been tried in patients seeking treatment. However, the results are unsatisfactory and the pigmentation reverts back after discontinuation of treatment.

Bibliography

1. Pigmentary demarcation lines over the face. Somani VK, Razvi F, Sita VN. Indian J Dermatol Venereol Leprol 2004 Nov-Dec;70(6):336–41.

2. Pigmentary demarcation lines over the face. Malakar S, Dhar S. Dermatology 2000;200(1):85–6.

2. RARE DISORDERS

PIGMENTED CONTACT DERMATITIS

Synonym: Melanodermatitis toxica, pigmented cosmetic dermatitis, female facial melanosis, Riehl's melanosis.

Pigmented contact dermatitis (PCD) is a non-eczematous variant of contact dermatitis. It was firstly described by Osmundsen, a Danish dermatologist, in 1970. He identified sentisation to 'spyrazoline', a component of optical whitener as the cause of an epidemic of melanosis in Copenhagen.

It can be caused by fragrances, nickel, dyes and cosmetics and thus is common condition which is misdiagnosed by most primary and tertiary care physicians.

Clinical Features

PCD is characterized by reticulate slate-gray or brown pigmentation caused by frequent and repeated contact with very small amounts of the contact sensitizer, mainly in textiles, fragrances or washing materials (Fig. 4.13a to c). A few patients may have subtle signs of dermatitis in the form of erythema and pruritus. Site of involvement depends on the allergen responsible with face being the commonest site. Axillae and anterior aspect of thigh may be affected in cases of dress dermatitis.

Pigmented cosmetic contact dermatitis (PCCD) is a variant of PCD proposed by Nakayama et al. The only difference being the causative allergens are the many ingredients in cosmetics such as fragrances (e.g. benzyl salicylate, cinnamic derivative, balsam of Peru), pigments, coal tar dyes and lanolin applied to the sites affected. Reihl's melanosis is considered synonymous with

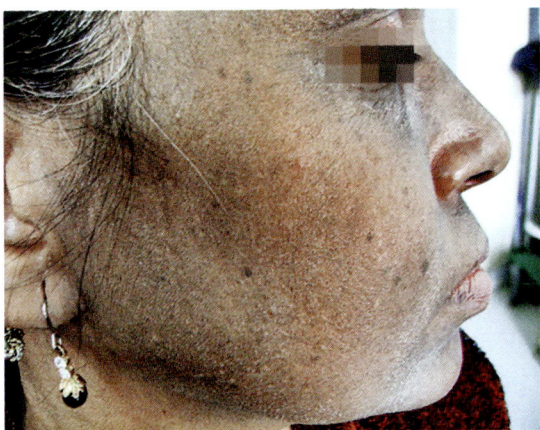

Fig. 4.13a: A case of toxic melanosis in a female. The possible cause is PPD which is a component of hair dye (chemical and so-called herbal dye)

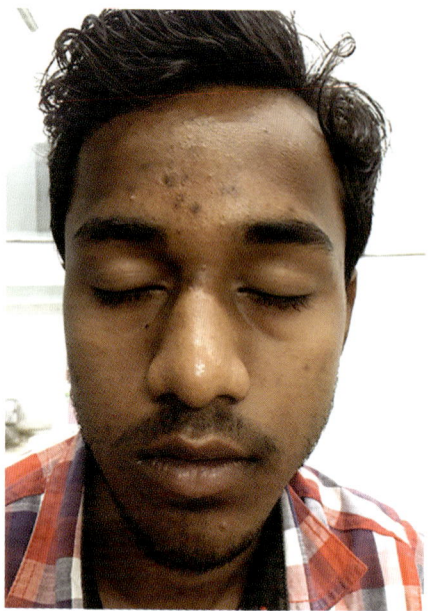

Fig. 4.13b: Toxic melanoderma secondary to mustard oil application in a young male

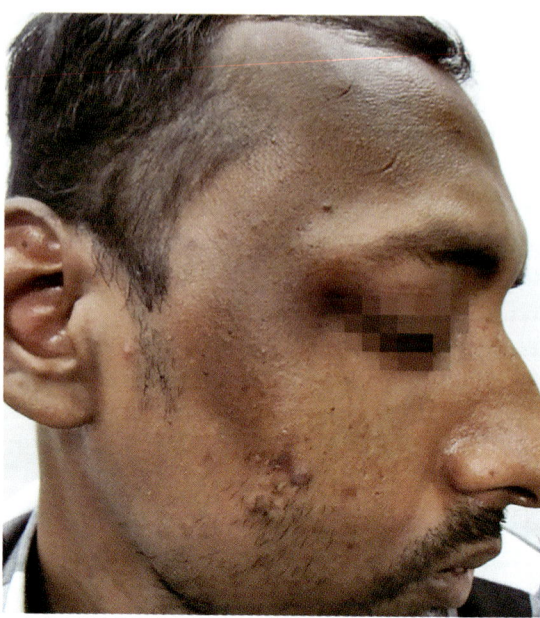

Fig. 4.13c: Pigmented contact dermatitis due to almond oil application over face

PCD with fragrances and chemicals in cosmetics being the allergen responsible. It was first described by Reihl in Vienna who observed grayish to brown pigmentation on the lateral aspect of face in several patients.

PCD usually occurs due to direct contact with allergens. Table 4.6 lists the common allergens implicated in PCD. In India, the commonest allergen causing PCD is kumkum, especially the red kumkum.

The exact mechanism of pigmentation in PCD is unknown. However, it has been suggested that the allergens responsible for this condition incite an inflammatory reaction around melanocytes due to their affinity for melanin. A few authors have suggested that Type IV hypersensitivity reaction at the basal layer causes pigmentary incontinence resulting in hyperpigmentation.

Table 4.6: List of allergens implicated in PCD	
Fragrances	Benzyl salicylate, benzyl alcohol, cinnamic alcohol, ylang-ylang oil, canaga oil, jasmine, synthetic sandalwood, lavender oil, geraniol, musk-ambrette, musk moskene, lemon oil and hydroxycitronellal
Textiles	Azo dyes, optical whiteners (Tinopal CH3566), Naphthol AS, Biocheck 60®, PPP-HB
Lipsticks	Diisostearyl malate, lanolin alcohol
Cosmetics	Phenyl salicylate, propolis, 2-bromo-2-nitropropane-1,3-diol (bronopol), Methyldibromo glutaronitrile (MDBGN)
Oils	Mustard and olive oil
Others	Potassium dichromate, 4-phenylenediamine base (PPD), colophony, balsam of Peru, paraben mix, sorbitan sesquioleate 5%, quaternium 15 (Dowicil 200), Ni sulfate, cobalt (II) chloride hexahydrate

Diagnosis/Investigations

Patch testing is of immense value in diagnosing PCD. Referral to dermatologist is advisable. The condition is difficult to diagnose and differentiate from lichen planus pigmentosus and ashy dermatoses and they may well be a continuum.

Treatment

In India, since there is very little control over the cosmetic industry, numerous OTC products containing the allergens abound with various 'herbal' and 'natural' tags. The use of expensive, so-called imported products, is no guarantee against the development of this problem. Thus, minimising the use of cosmetics to what has been tried previously and found safe is better than experimenting with new products. It is a good practice to ask the patient to use this list (Table 4.6) to scan the cosmetics as it is difficult to ensure that the patient stops all cometics and it is impossible for the doctor to remember the list!

On complete stopping of these agents resolution has been seen by Japanese dermatologist over 2–3 years. Oral HCQS and topical non-HQ based medications have been tried. Tretinoin should be scrupulously avoided as the irritation adds to the pigmentation, in Indian skin types.

Bibliography

Nakayama H, Matsuo S, Hayakawa K, Takashi K, Shigematsu T, Ota S. Pigmented cosmetic dermatitis. Int J Dermato 1984; 23: 299–30.

LICHEN PLANUS PIGMENTOSUS

Bhutani et al. first described lichen planus pigmentosus in 1974. LPP, an uncommon variant of LP, is commonly found in young to middle-aged females adults with skin phototypes III–V, especially patients of Indian, Latin American or Middle Eastern origin.

The exact etiology of LPP is unknown. A number of agents like cosmetics including fragrances, hair dyes, and mustard oil have been incriminated as the predisposing factors. Other postulated agents include sunlight, hepatitis C virus, gold.

Clinical Features

The disease usually starts after the age of 30. Clinically, it presents as irregularly shaped or oval brown to gray-brown macules and patches in either sun-exposed areas (especially the forehead, temples and neck) or intertriginous zones with asymptomatic to mild pruritus or a burning sensation (Fig. 4.14a and b). The pigmentation can be diffuse, blotchy, reticulate or perifollicular and symmetrical in distribution. Early lesions with an erythematous border as seen in ashy dermatosis are not a feature of LPP, which helps to distinguish between these two conditions, even though it is uncommon.

Mucous membranes are usually spared. However, some patients may have LP-like lesions in oral cavity.

Investigations

Hepatitis C serology and skin biopsy. The histopathological changes consist of vacuolar degeneration of the basal layer along with a perivascular lymphohistiocytic infiltrate and the presence of melanophages in the dermis.

Diagnosis

It has to be differentiated from Ashy Dermatoses aka EDP. In LPP, lesions begin on the sun-exposed areas of the body (temple/preauricular area) and they progressively involve the trunk and flexures.

EDP involves the unexposed sites. It starts on the trunk and then proceeds to involve the neck, proximal extremities and rarely the face. The lesions are arranged in a 'fir tree'-like pattern on the trunk.

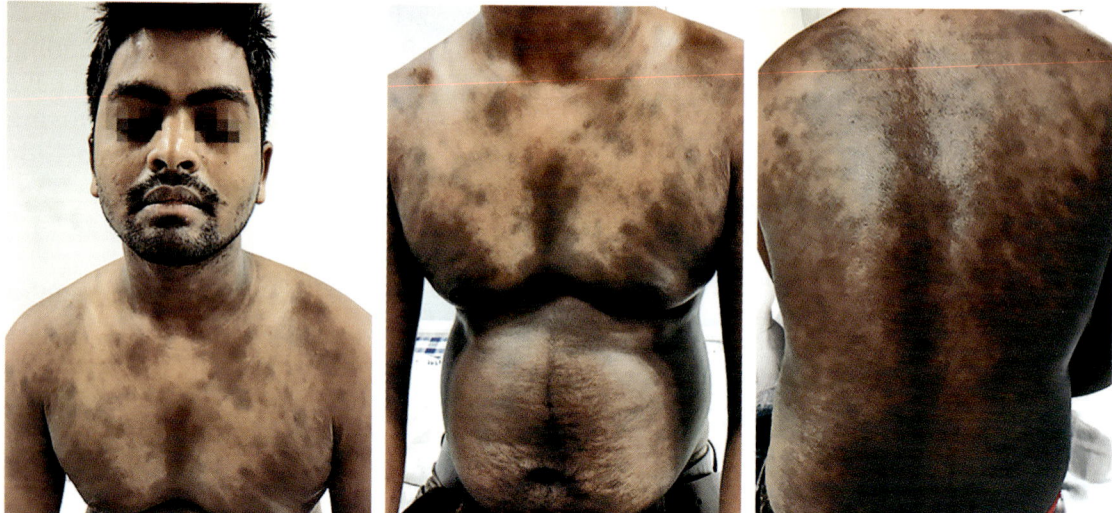

Fig. 4.14a: A young male with extensive lichen plans pigmentosus involving the face and trunk. The patient was started on dapsone along with sun protective measures

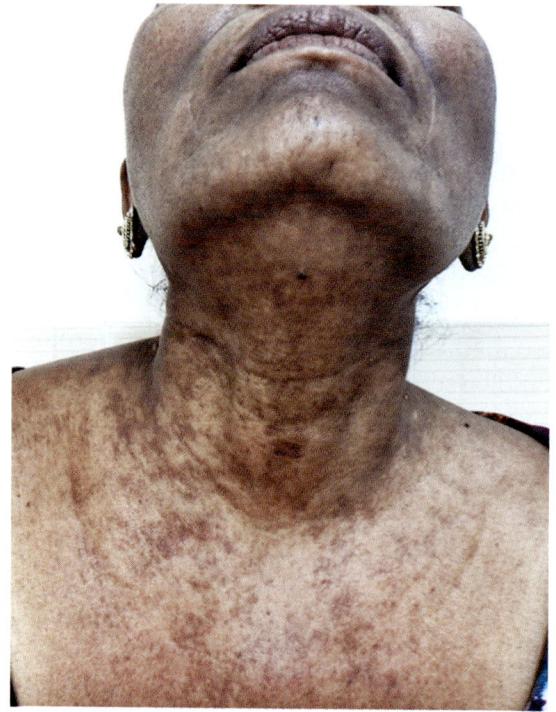

Fig. 4.14b: Lichen planus pigmentosus

Other differential diagnoses that should be considered include macular amyloidosis, pigmented contact dermatitis, drug-induced hyperpigmentation and post-inflammatory hyperpigmentation.

Treatment

The disease is insidious in onset and has a chronic course. The overview of the treatment modalities is given in Table 4.7.

Table 4.7: Overview of treatment of LPP

	Medical management	Cosmetic intervention	Laser/surgery
Topical	Mometasone cream once daily for 2 months Tacrolimus 0.1% twice daily for 4 months	Chemical peels	
Systemic	Clofazamine Dapsone Isotretinoin		
Level of care	**Primary** Use of sunscreen and sun avoidance	**Tertiary** Refer to dermatologist	**Tertiary** Refer to dermatologist

Bibliography

1. Al-Mutairi N, El-Khalawany M. Clinicopatholo-gical characteristics of lichen planus pigmentosus and its response to tacrolimus ointment: An open label, non-randomized, prospective study. J EurAcadDermatolVenereol 2010 May;24(5):535–40.

2. Bhutani LK, Bedi TR, Pandhi RK, Nayak NC. Lichen planus pigmentosus. Dermatologica 1974; 149: 43–50.

3. Breathnach SM. Lichen Planus and Lichenoid disorders. In: Burns T, Breathnach S, Cox N, Griffiths C, editors. Rook's Textbook of Der-matology, 8th edition. Oxford: Blackwell Science 2010, P. 41.13.

4. Kanwar AJ, Dogra S, Handa S, Parsad D, Radotra BD. A study of 124 Indian patients with lichen planus pigmentosus. ClinExpDermatol2003; 28:481–5.

POST-CHIKUNGUNYA HYPERPIGMENTATION

Chikungunya presents as fever, erythematous maculopapular rash and joint pains. Rarely, it may manifest as asymptomatic hyper-pigmented macules over the centrofacial area (Fig. 4.15) of face that is brownish-black or slate colored. It persists for about three to six months after infection. Melasma-like pigmentation and periorbital hyper-melanosis can also occur.

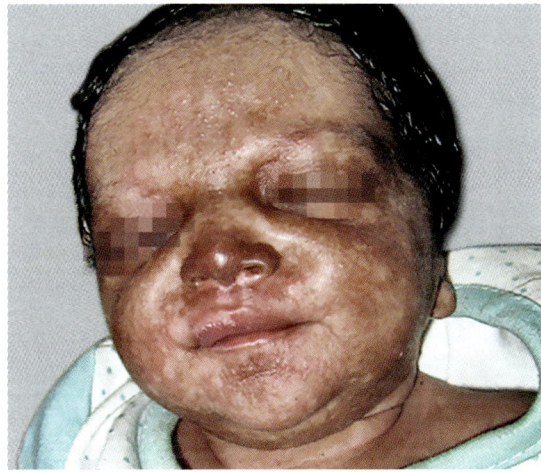

Fig. 4.15: A neonate with hyperpigmentation over face that occurred after chikungunya

POIKILODERMA OF CIVATTE (POC)

Poikiloderma refers to skin changes with thinning, increased pigmentation and dila-tion of the small blood vessels (telangiectasia).

In POC, the skin is red-brown with prominent hair follicles, affecting the neck and lateral cheeks, characteristically with sparing of the shaded area under the chin.

The cause is unknown, however, there is an association with UV exposure and it is more common in patients with fair skin. An additional theory is the photosensitising components of cosmetics and toiletries especially perfumes, although many doubt this link.

Refer to dermatologist for management.

Bibliography

Pigmentation Disorders. In. Sardana K, Garg VK, Mahajan S, eds. Diagnosis and Management of Skin Diseases: An Evidence Based Approach, Wolters Kluwer, LWW 2012, 1st edition.

NEVUS OF OTA

It is also known as oculodermal melanocytosis. It is a dermal melanocytic hamartoma that presents as bluish-brown patchy hyperpigmentation on the face along the first or second branches of the trigeminal nerve. It is more common in Asian females (Fig. 4.16a and b).

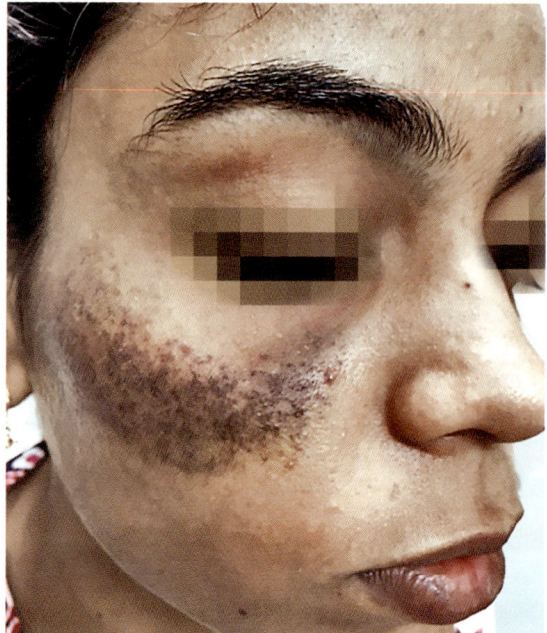

Fig. 4.16a: A female with nevus of Ota

Etiology

The etiopathogenesis of nevus of Ota is unknown. An increased number of melanocytes are seen in the involved skin. Several theories have been suggested for this which include dropping off of epidermal melanocytes and reactivation of latent dermal melanocytes by UV radiation, hormonal changes or dermal inflammation.

Clinical Features

Lesions are usually present at birth or occur during the first year of life. It can also appear around puberty.

The condition is characterized by unilateral, irregular, patchy bluish gray to brown hyperpigmentation in the periorbital region, temple, malar prominence, nose and forehead. Ocular involvement occurs in 60% of cases in the form of scleral and conjunctival pigmentation. Rarely, bilateral lesions can occur.

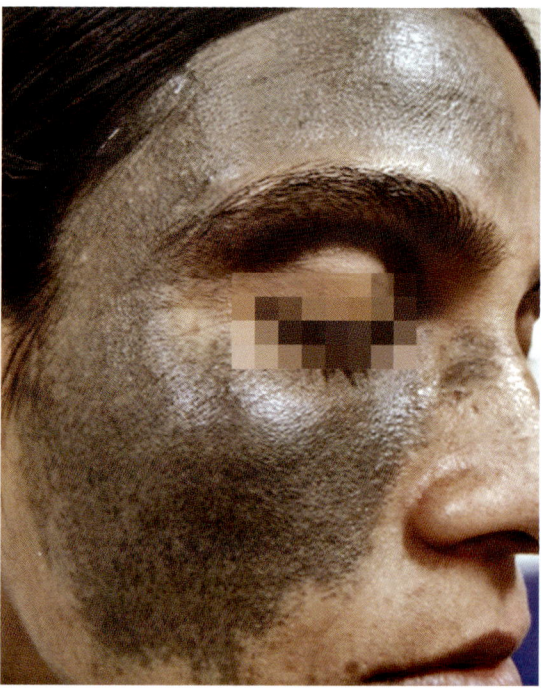

Fig. 4.16b: A female with nevus of Ota

Diagnosis

Diagnosis can be confirmed by histopathology that reveals elongated dendritic melanocytes in large numbers scattered among the collagen fibres in superficial dermis.

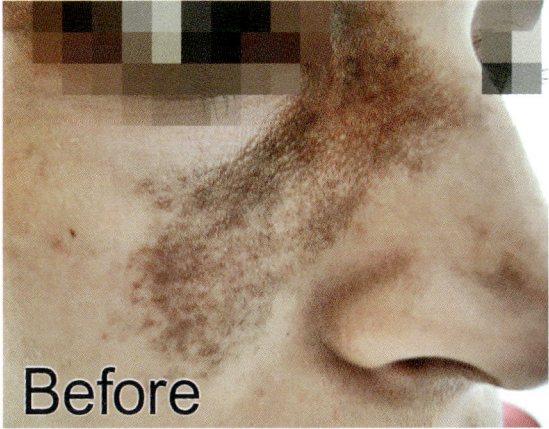 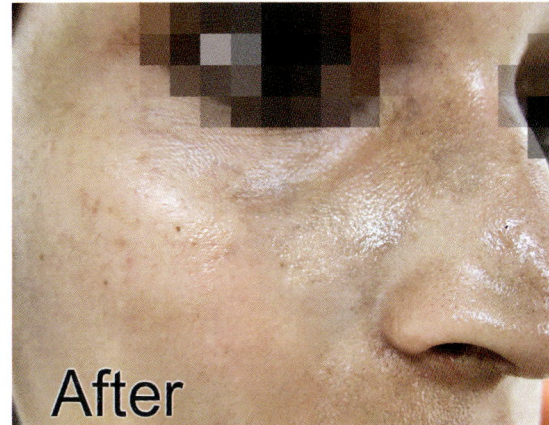

Before

After

Fig. 4.16c: Female with a brown-colored nevus of Ota (left) and after 4 sittings of Qs Nd:YAG (1064) laser

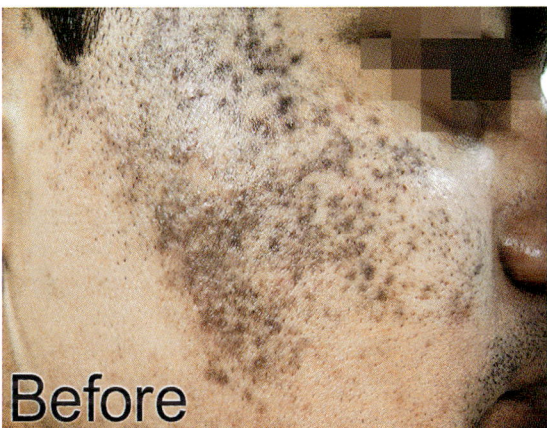 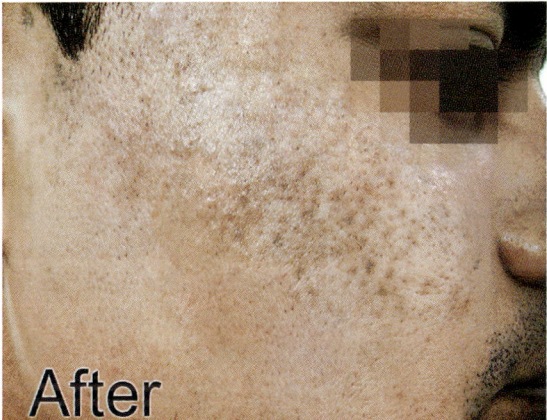

Before

After

Fig. 4.16d: Male patient with a blue-colored nevus of Ota (left) and after 12 sittings of Qs Nd:YAG (1064) laser

Treatment

Q-switched lasers are the mainstay of treatment but results depend on the age of the patient and the depth of pigmentation (Fig. 4.16c and d).

Complications

Malignant transformation, though rare, has been described hence patients should be kept under follow-up.

EXOGENOUS OCHRONOSIS (EO)

EO is a cutaneous disorder that occurs due to use of chemical substances on the face. It is synonymous with endogenous ochronosis or alkaptonuric ochronosis.

Such treatment may have been prescribed or used without the knowledge of a health professional.

Clinical Findings

EO is characterized by the presence of asymptomatic bilaterally symmetrical speckled blue black to gray brown macules (Fig. 4.17a and b) on the face mainly the malar areas, lower cheeks, temples and neck. Papular and nodular lesions may occur. It can also affect the cartilage of ear and sclera of eyes. In early stages, it resembles melasma.

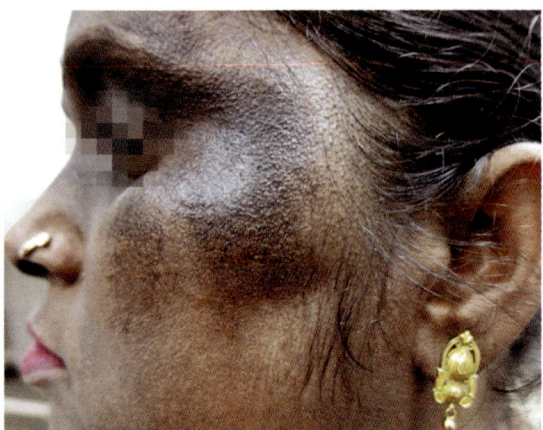

Fig. 4.17a: Ochronosis due to use of combination fairness creams

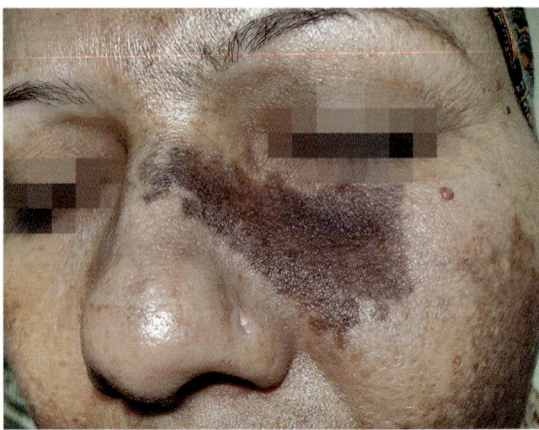

Fig. 4.17b: A case of localized ochronosis due to use of HQ 4% cream

Etiology

EO most commonly occurs due to use of topical hydroquinone (used as a skin lightening agent) but has also been described with use of phenol, resorcinol, quinine, mercury, picric acid and oral antimalarials. Various factors that predispose to EO are sunexposure, prolonged use of HQ over a larger area or in large quantity. The lesions develop gradually over 6 months to 3 years.

The exact pathogenesis is unknown but according to the most accepted hypothesis, there is competitive inhibition of the enzyme homogentistic oxidase by hydroquinone leading to accumulation of homogentistic acid and its metabolic products that polymerise to form the ochronotic pigment in the papillary dermis. This causes the clinical appearance of hyperpigmentation.

Diagnosis

It requires a high index of suspicion as the condition resembles melasma in early stages. Treatment with HQ can further aggravate the condition. Wood's lamp examination, dermoscopy and reflectance confocal microscopy are non-invasive tools that help in diagnosis.

Histopathology remains the gold standard for diagnosis. It is characterized by presence of ochre-colored, banana-shaped fibbers in the dermis.

Treatment

Exogenous ochronosis is difficult to treat. The most important thing is to stop the offending agent.

Various treatment modalities that have been tried are:

- *Sunscreens:* These should be used along with adequate sun protection measures.
- *Topical agents:* Retinoic acid, glycolic acid, vitamin C.
- *Procedural treatment:* Chemical peeling (with glycolic acid, tricarboxylic acid), dermabrasion, lasers (CO_2, Q-switched alexandrite 755 nm).

Bibliography

Pigmentation Disorders. In Sardana K, Garg VK, Mahajan S, eds. Diagnosis and Management of Skin Diseases: An Evidence Based Approach, Wolters Kluwer, LWW 2012, 1st edition.

Non-Melanin Pigmentation

Pooja Arora Mrig

Non-melanin pigmentation can be exogenous or endogenous. Endogenous causes include substances produced in the body in more than physiologic amount or in abnormal amount that get deposited in various body parts. Exogenous causes include chemicals and drugs deposited in the skin due to occupational exposure or as medication. The causes of non-melanin pigmentation are summarized in Table 5.1.

ENDOGENOUS PIGMENTATION

Cutaneous Hemosiderosis

Hemosiderin is a brown iron-binding pigment found within macrocytes. Deposition of hemosiderin causes brownish pigmentation in the skin by the following mechanisms:

- Local destruction of red blood cells leading to deposition of hemosiderin
- Stimulation of melanogenesis by hemosiderin
- Dermal pigmentation due to pigment incontinence

Clinical features depend on the underlying mechanism causing the condition.

Hypostatic Hemosiderosis

This occurs in patients with chronic venous hypertension where there is leakage of blood

Table 5.1: Causes of non-melanin pigmentation			
Endogenous		*Exogenous*	
Cutaneous hemosiderosis	Traumatic Hypostatic Capillaritis Congenital hemolytic anemia Hemochromatosis Dermatitis	Metals	Argyria Arsenic Bismuth Chrysiasis Mercury
Jaundice and bronze baby syndrome		Drugs	
Carotenoderma		Tattoos	
Ochronosis		Exogenous ochronosis	

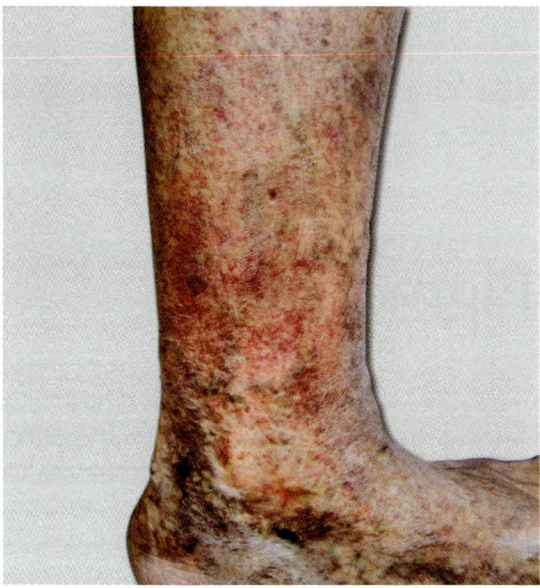

Fig. 5.1: A case of pigmented purpuric dermatosis where the pigmentation is consequent to capillary fragility and consequent hemosiderin deposition in the dermis

cells into extravascular spaces. Macrophages cause breakdown of red blood cells which leads to release of iron that combines with hemosiderin within macrocytes (Fig. 5.1).

Jaundice

Jaundice refers to yellowish discoloration of skin, eyes and mucous membranes due to deposition of bile pigments.

It occurs due to accumulation of bilirubin in tissues. Due to the high affinity of bilirubin for elastic tissues, the yellowish color is first seen in the sclerae. The color can vary depending on the presence of biliverdin which gives a greenish hue. Jaundice of long duration can give rise to bronze discoloration of skin.

Jaundice should be differentiated from carotenemia (described below).

Bronze Baby Syndrome (BBS)

Phototherapy in children with jaundice can cause brown-bronze pigmentation of skin, mucosae and urine. It occurs due to:

- Abnormal accumulation of bilirubin photoisomers.
- Abnormal hepatic function leading to accumulation of copper porphyrin complexes that cause brown pigmentation.
- Abnormal accumulation of biliverdin.

BBS should be differentiated from gray baby syndrome seen in neonates due to high doses of chloramphenicol.

No treatment is required as BBS disappears after stopping phototherapy. However, the underlying liver disease should be identified and treated.

Carotenoderma (Xanthoderma)

Carotenemia refers to excessive carotenoids in the blood which can result in carotenoderma which is the excessive carotene in skin leading to yellowish discoloration.

Carotenoids are yellow-colored, lipid-soluble compounds found in vegetables and fruits. These include alpha and beta carotene, lycopene, lutein, canthazanthin, etc. These are normal part of our diet and contribute to normal color of skin.

Primary carotenoderma occurs due to excessive intake of foods containing carotene, e.g. orange, carrots, pumpkin, etc. It is also seen in young children given large amounts of commercial infant food preparations and in food faddists who consume food stuffs with high carotene content.

Secondary carotenoderma occurs in conditions such as diabetes, hyperlipidemia, hypothyroidism, nephritis and inborn errors of metabolism. It occurs in patients on oral supplements of beta carotene (exceeding 30 mg daily).

Clinical Features

There is yellowish discoloration of skin especially in areas where horny layer is thickened such as palms and soles (Fig. 5.2). It is also more prominent in areas where there is abundant subcutaneous fat. The

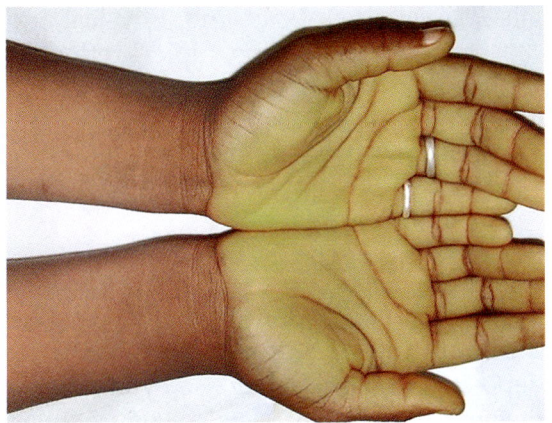

Fig. 5.2: A depiction of carotenemia with marked accentuation on the palms

sclera and mucous membranes are not affected. Yellow sclera is classically seen in jaundice.

Serum beta carotene levels are elevated by three to four times the normal level.

Serum levels of carotene come back to normal after dietary restriction. However, yellow color may persist for a few months.

Ochronosis

Ochronosis is derived from the word "ochre" which means yellowish discoloration. It can be exogenous or endogenous.

Endogenous Ochronosis

Endogenous ochronosis is the pigmentation that occurs in skin in patients with alkaptonuria which is a rare metabolic disease.

Pathophysiology: In alkaptonuria, there is total deficiency of enzyme homogentisic acid oxidase. Homogentisic acid is a part of the metabolic pathway of amino acids phenylalanine and tyrosine. Deficiency of this enzyme leads to accumulation of homogentisic acid in the body especially the skin, skeletal system, eyes and cardiovascular system. Pigmentation occurs in 75% of patients with alkaptonuria and is more common in darkly pigmented skin.

Clinical features: There is bluish discoloration of cartilage of the ear cartilage which may be accompanied by blackened discoloration of earwax. There is pigmentation of sclera, cornea, conjunctiva and eyelids. There is brownish pigmentation over face; more prominent over malar and axillary regions where there are greater number of sweat glands. Neck and trunk may be involved. Palmar and plantar skin may show bluish black vesicles or papules due to friction movements.

Differential diagnosis: Facial pigmentation should be differentiated from other causes of pigmentation like porphyria cutanea tarda, Addison's disease, hemochromatosis and drug-induced pigmentation.

Investigations: The diagnosis is made based on history and evaluation of homogentisic acid in urine. The latter is the gold standard of diagnosis.

Management: There is no definitive treatment. Ascorbic acid (1 g/day), nitisinone and a protein restricted diet have been tried with beneficial effects.

Exogenous Ochronosis

It is the blue black pigmentation of skin due to long-term application of topical skin lightening creams containing hydroquinone (Fig. 5.3). It can also occur due to contact with phenol or resorcinol.

Pathophysiology: There is inhibition of homogentisic oxidase leading to accumulation of homogentisic acid which polymerises to form ochre (brownish-yellow) pigment in the papillary dermis.

Both endogenous and exogenous ochronoses are histologically characterized by

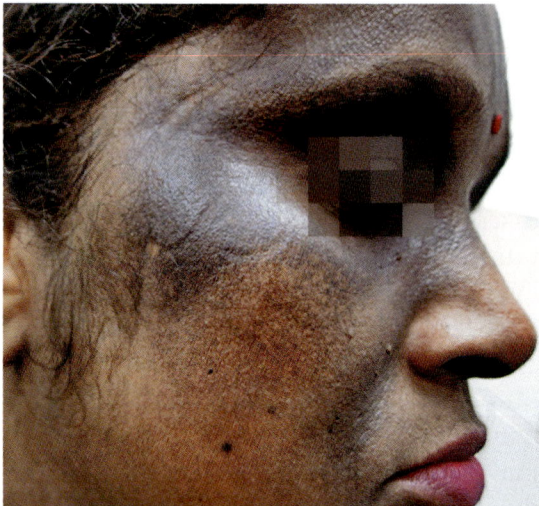

Fig. 5.3: Ochronosis in a female patient using a triple combination cream for melasma

comma- or banana-shaped ochronotic collagen bundles in dermis. Although the condition is more likely to occur at concentrations higher than 3% for prolonged periods of time (>6 months), it can also occur with concentration of 2% or less.

Clinical features: It is characterized by gray-brown or blue-black macules over areas of contact with hydroquinone. Unlike endogenous ochronosis, it is not associated with pigmentation of cartilage, sclerae or conjunctiva. There are no systemic features.

Differential diagnosis: The condition should be differentiated from other causes of facial pigmentation (mentioned above).

Investigations: The condition is diagnosed by patient history. Wood's lamp examination and dermoscopy may aide in diagnosis. Histopathology remains the gold standard in the diagnosis of exogenous ochronosis.

Treatment

i. *Non-pharmacological measures:* Stop further use of offending agents, strict sun protection.

ii. *Pharmacological measures:* Physical and chemical sunscreens, topical retinoids, glycolic acid, oral antioxidants.

iii. *Procedural treatments:* Chemical peeling with glycolic acid, dermabrasion, CO_2 laser, Q-switched Nd:YAG laser.

EXOGENOUS PIGMENTATION

Various chemicals and drugs can produce discoloration of skin not only by being deposited in the skin but also by increasing melanin in the skin. Metals such as silver, gold, mercury and bismuth can accumulate in the skin and cause severe disfiguring pigmentation (Table 5.2).

Drug-induced Hyperpigmentation

Hyperpigmentation can be induced by a variety of drugs. Several mechanisms have been postulated for drug-induced skin pigmentation. These include:

i. Increased melanin synthesis
ii. Deposition of drug-related material
iii. Increased lipofuscin synthesis
iv. Post-inflammatory hyperpigmentation

A few common drugs and the type of pigmentation are mentioned in Table 5.3.

Disease Course

Pigmentation usually disappears after discontinuation of causative drug. In a few patients, it may persist even after discontinuation.

Treatment

• Discontinuation of drug
• Sun protection
• Laser therapy for residual lesions

Tattoos

Tattoo is actually appearance of color through epidermis of the ink located in dermis. The process of tattooing involves dipping of needles into various inks. In older

Table 5.2: Metals associated with hyperpigmentation

Metal	Pattern of pigmentation
Silver (argyria)	Slate-gray pigmentation that appears many years later. Most apparent in sun-exposed areas of skin, especially forehead, nose and hands. Sclerae, nails and mucous membranes may be hyper-pigmented (Fig. 5.4).
Arsenic	Diffuse pigmentation more prominent on the trunk. There are macular areas of depigmentation within areas of hyper-pigmentation called "raindrop" appearance (Fig. 5.5). Associated features—arsenical keratosis which is bilateral thickening of palms and soles
Bismuth	Diffuse gray pigmentation resembling argyria. Also involves sclera and oral/vaginal mucous membrane. Characteristic blue-black line is seen at gingival margin. Hydrogen sulfide is formed by bacteria in the mouth reacts with bismuth deposited in the mucosa leading to this blue-black line
Chrysiasis and chrysoderma	Pigmentation of the skin due to parenteral administration of gold salts

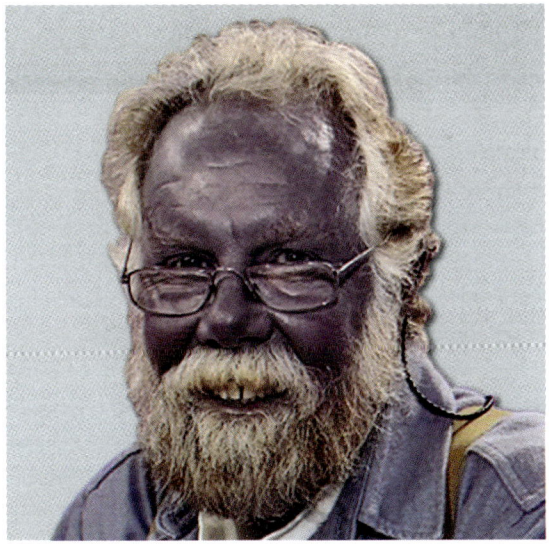

Fig. 5.4: This is an image of Mr Karason who shot to Internet fame several years ago for the blue color of his skin, which was a side effect of using a silver compound for more than a decade to treat a bad case of dermatitis on his face. This was colloidal silver a compound that is again being used in India to counteract various disorders in certain high end patients

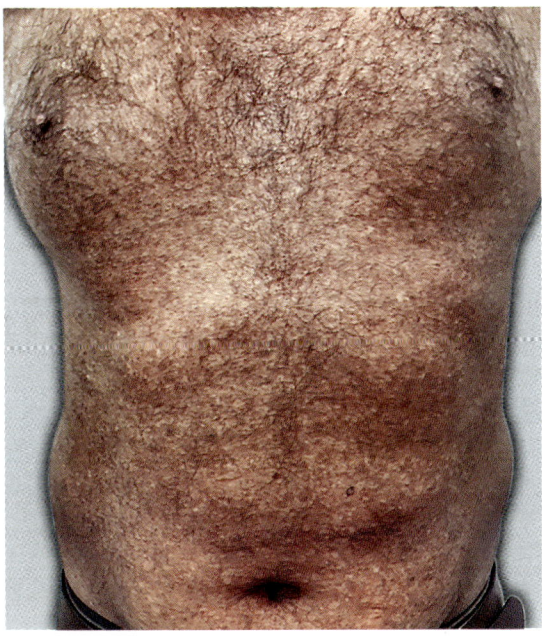

Fig. 5.5: A patient with "raindrop" pigmentation after arsenic intoxication due to consumption of ayurvedic medication containing arsenic

times, the pigment was introduced through a puncture wound with sharp instrument. Nowadays, electrical tattoo device injects ink particles from the epidermis to a constant depth (usually 1 mm) below the dermo-epidermal junction. The risk of unsterile tattoo technique includes transmission of various pathogens, i.e. hepatitis B and C, syphilis, HIV.

Table 5.3: Common drugs associated with pigmentation	
Drug	*Type of pigmentation*
Antimalarial drugs	Bluish-gray pigmentation on sun-exposed areas, nail beds, oral mucosa, bleaching of hair
Clofazimine	Initially red, later violaceous brown, most noticeable on lesional skin of leprosy (Fig. 5.6)
Cytotoxic drugs	Caused by busulphan, cyclophosphamide, bleomycin, fluorouracil, methotrexate May be localized/diffuse, may affect all parts of skin including mucous membranes, hair and nails (Fig. 5.7)
Phenytoin	Melasma-like pigmentation
Chlorpromazine	Blue-gray pigmentation of sun-exposed areas of skin
Tetracycline	Commonly with minocycline, well-circumscribed blue-gray macules located in areas of acne scars, sites of previous inflammation, sun-exposed areas, lower lip
Amiodarone	Slate-gray or purple discoloration of sun-exposed skin especially face with prominent involvement of nose

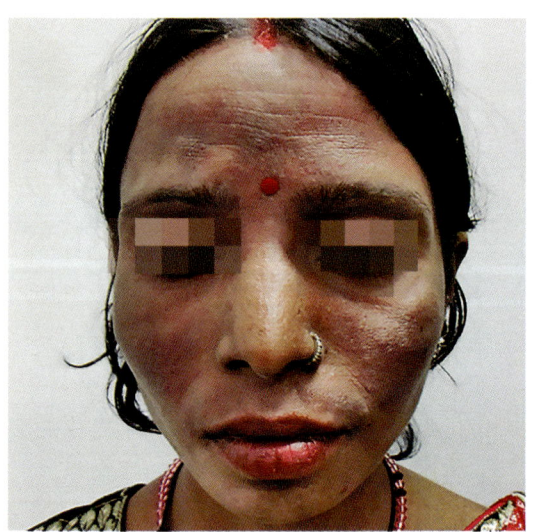

Fig. 5.6: Clofazimine-induced pigmentation over face in a patient on multidrug therapy for leprosy. Note the reddish-brown color of lesions

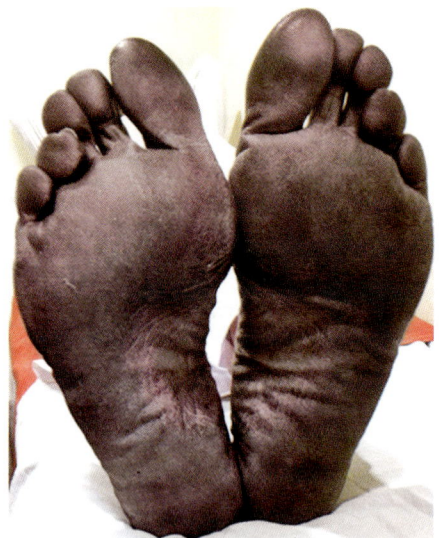

Fig. 5.7: Epirubicin-induced hyperpigmentation of soles

Types of Tattoos

Five different types of tattoos have been described in literature namely amateur, professional, cosmetic, medical and traumatic.

i. *Amateur tattoos:* These are made arbitrarily with devices such as tattoo gun, guitar string, battery and ink pens using charcoal and soot. These tattoos are usually light and easily removed because content used is organic ink.

ii. *Professional tattoos:* These tattoos are made by expert tattooists who have expertise in their field. In these tattoos, special inks such as metal oxide and iron oxide are used. These last for decades since tattoo ink is placed adequately deep and densely in the skin. These tattoos are harder to clear even with lasers.

iii. *Cosmetic tattoos:* These have become increasingly popular for natural pigmentation of areola after breast reconstruction and to simulate natural pigmentation on eyes and on cheek using colored dyes such as black, brown and pink.

iv. *Medical tattoos:* These are becoming popular as they provide information about the proper location for repeated radiotherapy and also for marking of areola in breast reconstruction. Surprisingly, "amalgam tattoo" may be acquired because of trauma or exposure to various metals used in dentistry. Tattooing has also been used in medical information transmission, i.e. blood group and in medical conditions such as those suffering from viral disease. Further, tattooing of vitiligo patches has also been described in medical literature.

v. *Traumatic tattoos:* These have been described after superficial abrasions which are contaminated with chemically inert particles. Wounds after bullet injury may introduce pigmented particles which results in pigmentation/tattooing of skin.

Additionally, a distinctive occupational mark in coalminers (collier's stripes) which are bluish-gray and linear or angular stripes develop at the site of abrasions, i.e. forehead, bridge of the nose, wrists and elbows. The particles of dust up to 100 μm in diameter when examined histologically are seen in the dermis and are specially grouped around blood vessel.

Technique of Tattooing

In case of professional tattoos, hand-held device, powered by low voltage direct current, holds solid needles placed singly or in groups of up to fourteen oscillating bars. The needles are dipped into colored inks and then moved across skin in desired pattern, penetrating rapidly and vertically 0.5–2.0 mm into the skin, depositing the pigment into dermis. Amateur tattooist often does it this way using handheld needles wound round with thread to prevent deep penetration. Other instruments used may be pencils, pens and straight pins.

Tattoo Ink

Various types of tattoo ink have been used and are depicted in Table 5.4.

Table 5.4: Various types of tattoo ink and their composition	
Colour of ink	*Composition*
Black	Carbon, iron oxide, logwood
Blue	Cobalt aluminate (azure blue)
Green	Chrome oxide, malachite green, lead chromate, ferro-ferric cyanide, curcumin green, phthalocyanide dyes
Red	Mercury sulfide (cinnabar), cadmium selenide (cadmium red), sienna ochre (ferric hydrate, ferric sulfate)
Violet	Manganese violet white
Yellow	Cadmium sulfide (cadmium yellow), ochre
White	Titanium oxide, zinc oxide
Brown	Ochre
Flesh	Iron oxides (variants of ochre)

Tattoo Reactions

Tattoo reactions can be divided into three main categories: Inflammatory, infectious, and neoplastic. Inflammatory manifestations include focal edema, pruritus, papules, or nodules at the tattoo site (Fig. 5.8a to c). Histologically, they can be classified as lichenoid, eczematoid, foreign body, granulomatous, and sarcoidal. Less commonly, psoriasiform, morpheaform, and vasculitic reactions have also been reported.

The infectious reactions may occur due to bacterial, viral or mycotic infections and they can appear as superficial or deep skin involvement.

Rarely, neoplastic complications such as keratoacanthoma, squamous cell and basal

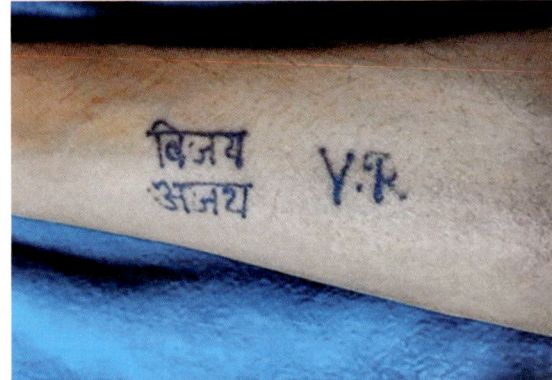

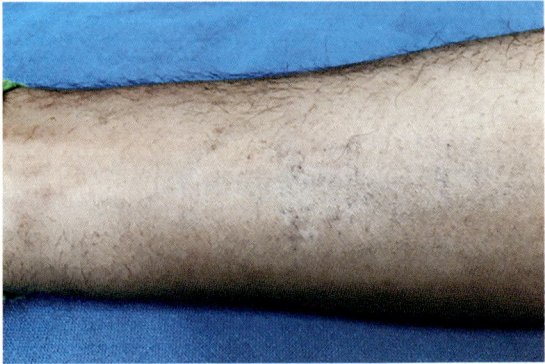

Fig. 5.8c: Patient with amateur tattoo treated with combination of CO_2 laser followed by Nd:YAG laser

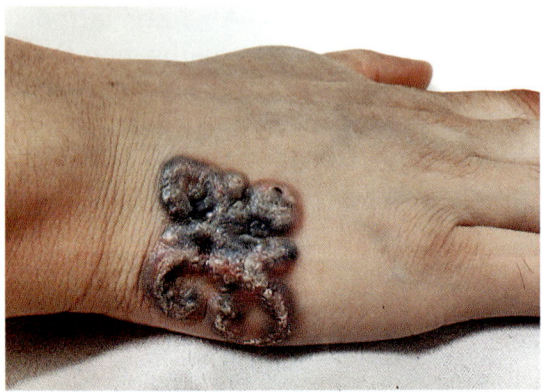

Fig. 5.8a: Lichenoid reaction to tattoo

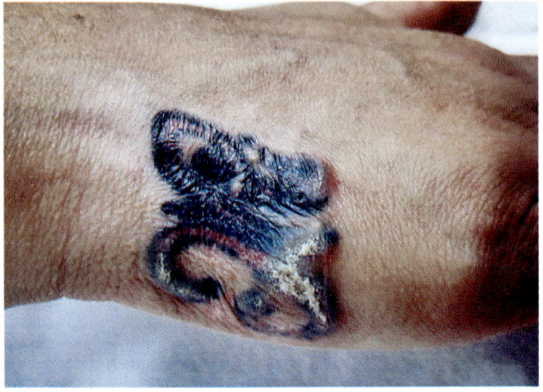

Fig. 5.8b: Response to treatment (flattening of lesion) after intralesional triamcinolone

cell carcinoma, leiomyosarcoma, and melanoma have been documented with tattoo pigments.

The most frequent tattoo reaction is the allergic contact dermatitis due to delayed hypersensitivity reaction to different pigments contained in the tattoos. The main pigment causing allergic reaction is red, due to the presence of mercury and its sulfides. However, nowadays, most reactions are not due to the traditional presence of mercury sulfides, but due to new organic pigments (e.g. Pigment Red 181 and Pigment Red 170). Blue, green, and black tattoos are a less frequent cause of allergic contact dermatitis. Actually allergy reactions to temporary henna tattoos due to the paraphenylenediamine (PPD) are very common due to prior exposure to PPD in hair dyes.

Tattoo Removal

The presence of tattoos may be considered highly inappropriate in certain situations and may affect interpersonal relationships and employment opportunities. There are many indications for tattoo removal such as

i. Cosmetic: Tattoo design may later on be disliked, its anatomical placement may be wrong and also for removal of mismatched color after vitiligo surgery.

ii. Medical: Such as hypersensitivity to tattoo pigment, removal of accidental tattoos of gunshot injury or vehicular accident, or when used as guideline tattoo marking the area for radiotherapy.

iii. Others such as impediment for professional employment or impairment, for a change or advancement in job.

Tattoos can be removed by various methods such as counter-tattooing, chemical methods, electro-surgery/radiosurgery, cryosurgery, dermabrasion alone or with tannic acid/silver nitrate/urea, surgical excision, infrared coagulator and various lasers.

Various lasers used for tattoo removal include the ablative lasers (CO_2 laser and argon laser) and non-ablative lasers (Q-switched Nd: YAG, ruby and alexandrite laser).

Bibliography

1. Bolognia JL, Jorizzo JJ. Schaffer JV. Dermatology. 3rd ed. London: Elsevier. 2012. Chapter 67 Disorders of Hyperpigmentation; p. 1049–1074.

2. Geel NV, Speeckaert R. Acquired Pigmentary Disorders. In: Griffith CEM, Barker J, Bleiker T, Chalmers R, Creamer D editors. Rook's Text Book of Dermatology. 9th ed. United Kingdom (UK): John Wiley & Sons publication; 2016.p.88.47–54.

3. Goldsmith LA, Katz SI, Gilchrest BA, Paller AS, Leffell DA, Wolff K. Fitzpatrick's Dermatology In General Medicine. 8th ed. New York: McGraw-Hill Medical, 2012. Chapter 75. Hypomelanoses and Hypermelanoses; p. 804–826.

Pigmented Skin Tumors

Aastha Gupta

Pigmented skin tumors are heterogeneous entities classified pathogenetically into melanocytic and non-melanocytic tumors. The differential diagnosis of pigmented skin tumors is illustrated in Figure 6.1a. The incidence of skin cancer is increasing worldwide and early diagnosis and treatment is crucial to prevent metastatic disease and mortality. Since only subtle differences exist between the benign and the malignant lesions, it is not always easy to establish a primary diagnosis based on clinical features, requiring histopathological evaluation in many cases. An algorithm is depicted which requires a dermatoscopic evaluation (Fig. 6.1b). Here we describe the commonly encountered pigmented neoplasms focusing on diagnosis and their management.

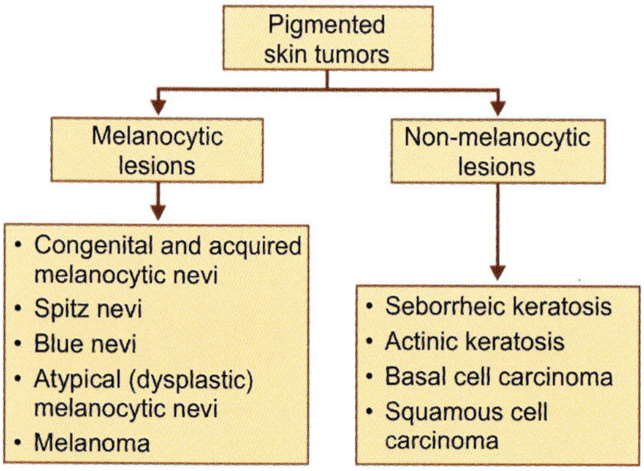

SEBORRHEIC KERATOSIS (SK)

Seborrheic keratosis is the most common benign epidermal neoplasm.

Epidemiology

The lesions typically appear during the fourth decade of life although they can develop during adolescence. They are more common in Caucasians and affect men and women with equal incidence. Familial predisposition with an autosomal dominant inheritance pattern with incomplete penetrance has been described for SK.

Clinical Features

They usually begin as solitary or multiple, well-circumscribed, dull, flat, tan to black patches with a waxy, verrucous, or "stuck on" appearance. Many lesions show the characteristic pseudohorn cysts which represent plugged follicular orifices and/or hyperkeratotic scales (Fig. 6.2). The lesions are seen on hair-bearing skin, sparing the mucosal surfaces and the palms and soles

Fig. 6.1a: Overview of pigmented skin tumors

and multiple lesions may be distributed along the Blaschko's lines or in a Christmas tree pattern. Although usually asymptomatic, inflamed or traumatized lesions may be pruritic, tender, crusted and, rarely pustular.

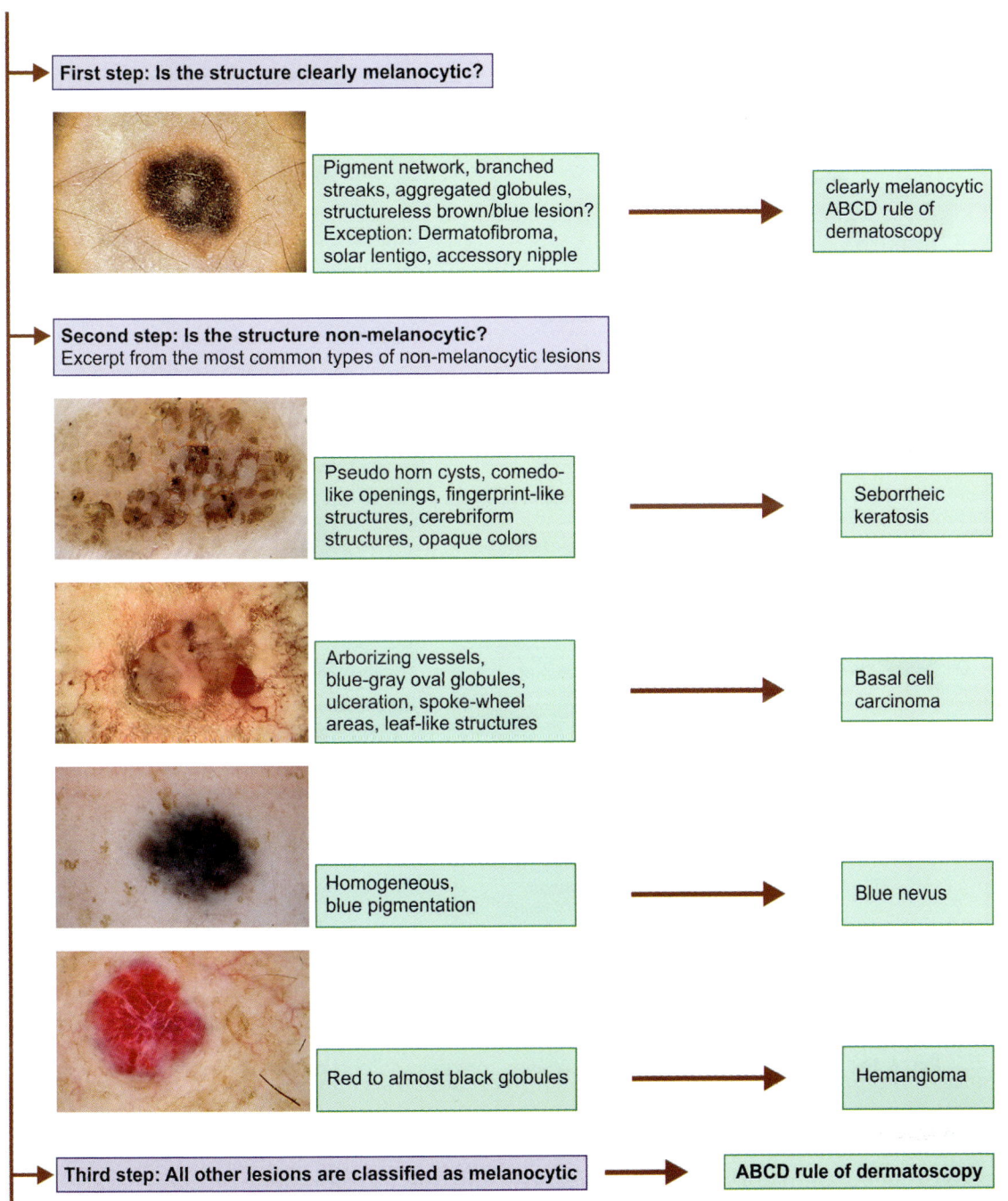

First step: Is the structure clearly melanocytic?

Pigment network, branched streaks, aggregated globules, structureless brown/blue lesion? Exception: Dermatofibroma, solar lentigo, accessory nipple → clearly melanocytic ABCD rule of dermatoscopy

Second step: Is the structure non-melanocytic?
Excerpt from the most common types of non-melanocytic lesions

Pseudo horn cysts, comedo-like openings, fingerprint-like structures, cerebriform structures, opaque colors → Seborrheic keratosis

Arborizing vessels, blue-gray oval globules, ulceration, spoke-wheel areas, leaf-like structures → Basal cell carcinoma

Homogeneous, blue pigmentation → Blue nevus

Red to almost black globules → Hemangioma

Third step: All other lesions are classified as melanocytic → ABCD rule of dermatoscopy

(Contd.)

| Fourth step: ABCD rule of dermatoscopy | Examples: |

A

Asymmetry:
Asymmetric in
one or two axis

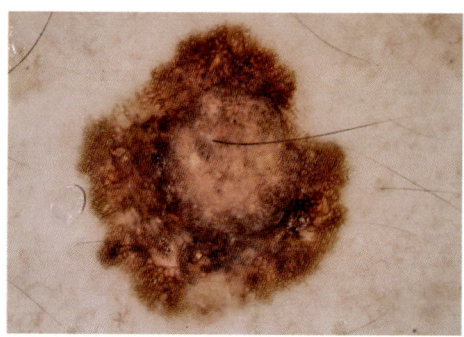

B

Border:
Irregular or
blurred

Asymmetrical lesion with atypical network, stripes, and dots with brown, gray, and blue colors. Image without polarization filter with immersion fluid and full lighting (4 LEDs).

C

Color:
Differently colored
pigmentation
Polychromatism
(white, red, light
brown, dark brown,
black, and blue-gray)

D

Dermatoscopic structure:
Pigment network—irregular mesh and/or pigmentation (1)
Clumps and globules—irregular size and distribution (2)
Branched strips—modified pigment network, abrupt discontinuation (3)
Strips—non-parallel, irregular strips (4)
Structureless areas—no recognisable structures (5), milky veil
Regression structures—whitish, scar-like depigmentation (6)
Atypical vascular patterns—irregular polymorphous vascular pattern (7), hairpin vessels (8), milky red areas (9)

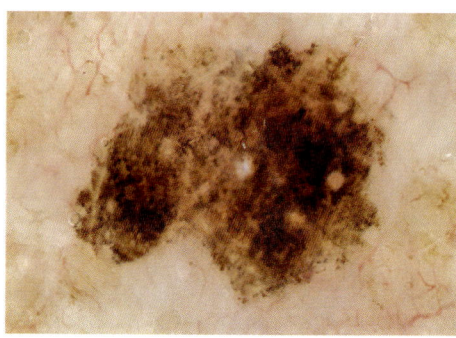

Asymmetric lesion with clumps, points, and a network of an invasive melanoma (<0.5 mm tumor thickness) with brown and gray colors. Image with polarization filter with immersion fluid and full lighting (4 LEDs).

If one or more of these criteria correspond to a pigment spot, a suspicious or malignant lesion may be involved.

Fig. 6.1b: Algorithm for differentiating between melanocytic and non-melanocytic skin tumors

Sign of Leser-Trélat, i.e. an abrupt "flare" of lesions is seen during pregnancy, coexisting inflammatory dermatoses (particularly erythroderma) and internal malignancy. Spontaneous regression is uncommon and rapidly growing, symptomatic, or unusual lesions should be biopsied to rule out the development of malignancies like basal cell carcinoma, squamous cell carcinoma, or melanoma. Dermatosis papulosa

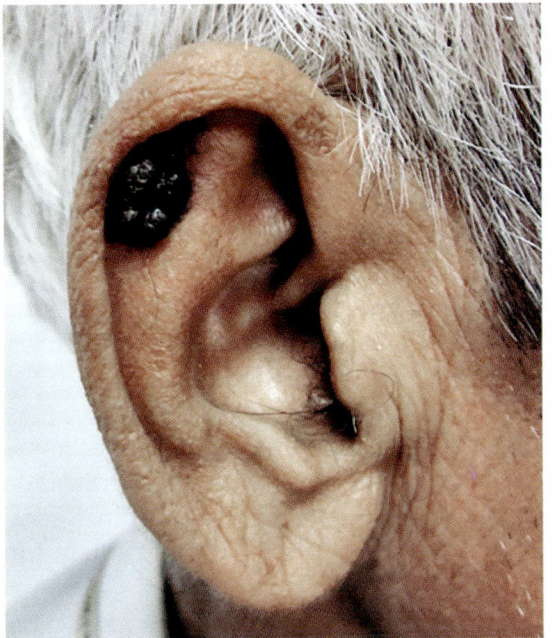

Fig. 6.2: Hyperpigmented verrucous papules on the pinna in an elderly male. Note the "stuck on" appearance

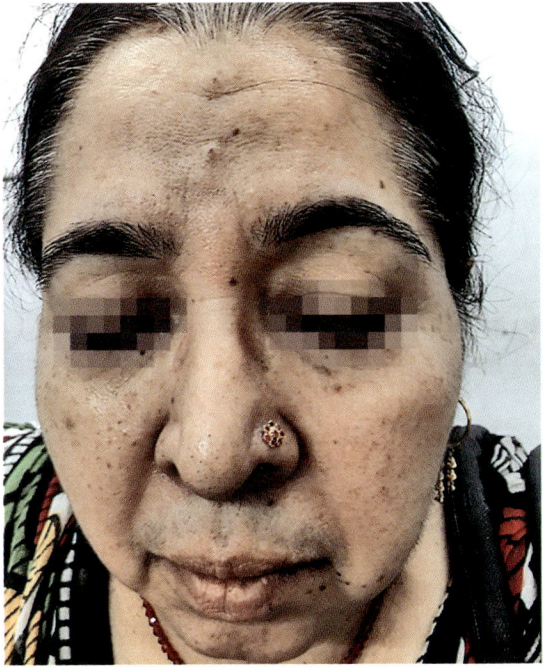

Fig. 6.3a: Dermatosis papulosa nigra: Multiple hyperpigmented papules over the face in a 50-year-old female. This is a clinical variant of SK

nigra (DPN) is a common clinical variant of SK (Fig. 6.3a).

A remarkably dark, flat, or thick seborrheic keratosis (Fig. 6.3b) may also be challenging in the differential diagnosis of various melanocytic tumors. This type of seborrheic keratosis has been called "melanoacanthoma".

Pathogenesis

Although the exact etiology of SK is unknown, genetics, sun exposure, and infection have all been implicated as possible factors. The higher prevalence of lesions on sun-exposed areas implies a possible causative role. Also, viral infection has also been implicated based on the clinical and histological similarities of SKs to warts and the infrequent detection of human papillomavirus (HPV) in these lesions.

Pathology

Hallmark histopathologic findings include acanthosis, papillomatosis, hyperkeratosis

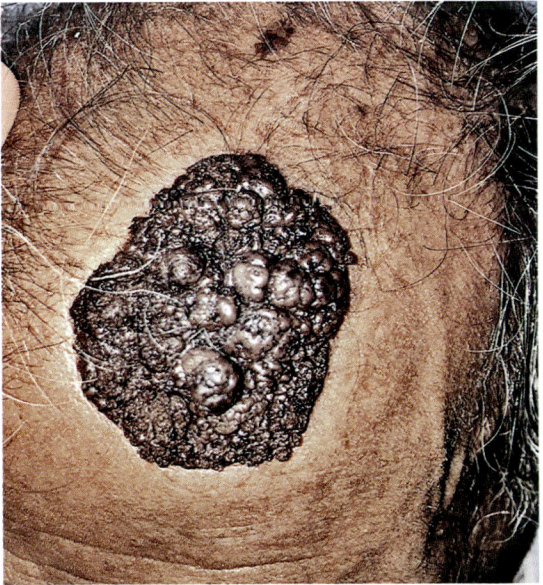

Fig. 6.3b: Melanoacathoma: This is the pigmented subtype of seborrheic keratosis

and the presence of pseudohorn cysts. Generally, the base of a SK lies on a flat horizontal plane flanked by normal epidermis called the "string" sign. Cytologic atypia is usually not seen.

Treatment

Treatment of asymptomatic SKs is mainly performed for cosmetic reasons. Lesions are usually removed by curettage, destruction or shave excision. The common methods of destruction include cryotherapy, electrodesiccation or laser vaporization (pulsed CO_2, erbium:YAG).

ACTINIC KERATOSES

Actinic keratoses (AKs) or solar keratoses are precancerous or premalignant lesions consisting of proliferations of cytologically abnormal keratinocytes that develop due to prolonged ultraviolet (UV) radiation exposure. They are one of the strongest predictors of subsequent development of melanoma or non-melanoma skin cancer (NMSC).

Epidemiology

AKs are most commonly found in fair-skinned individuals with the prevalence increasing with age and cumulative UV exposure. It is more common in males and in patients with immunosuppression and certain genetic syndromes, such as, albinism and xeroderma pigmentosum.

Clinical Features

The typical AK lesion is an erythematous, flat, rough, scaly papule with white to yellow scale varying in size from a few millimeters to several centimeters in diameter (Figs 6.4 and 6.5). They are most often found on sun-exposed areas of the body, such as the head and neck, forearms, and dorsal hands and are found against a background of photo-damaged skin with solar elastosis, dyspigmentation, lentigos and telangiectasias. Pruritus, bleeding, and crusting may be present but presence of pain, inflammation and ulceration are clues to the transition to SCC. The risk for malignant transformation of AK to SCC varies from less than 1 to 20%.

Pigmented AKs lack erythema and have a hyperpigmented or reticulated appearance. Clinical clues such as location on sun-exposed skin, background solar changes, and hyperkeratosis and dermoscopy or biopsy may be useful in these cases.

Pathogenesis

Although genetic and environmental factors may play a role in the development of AK, the most important factor is exposure to UV radiation, that is, sunlight exposure. UV radiation-induced somatic mutations in p53,

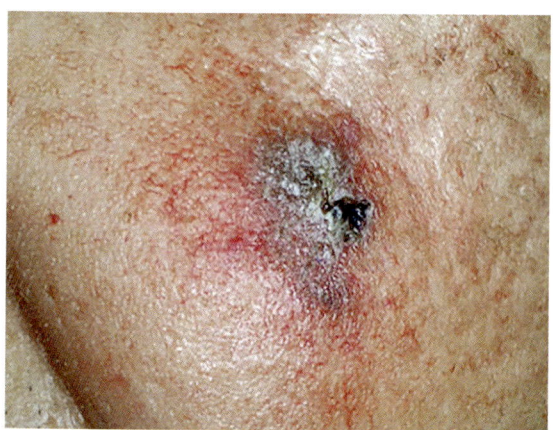 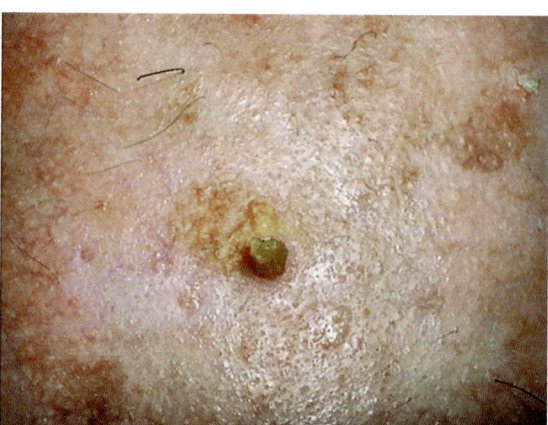

Fig. 6.4: Actinic keratoses on the side of the nose (left) and on the scalp

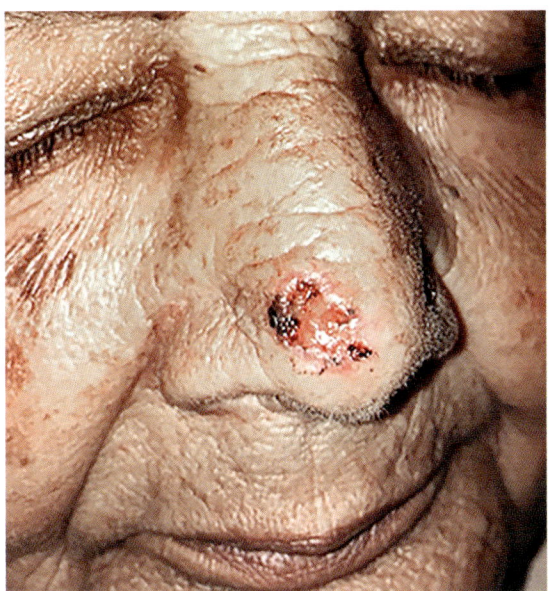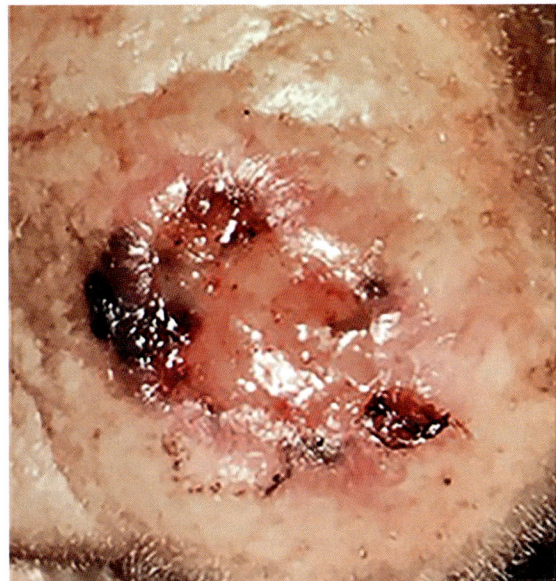

Fig. 6.5: Basal cell carcinoma: Shiny translucent papule with smooth surface and telangiectasias. Note the rolled out border

a tumor suppressor gene, play a pivotal role in the development of AKs and their progression into SCC.

Pathology

AK is characterized by atypical keratinocytic proliferation, displaying nuclear pleomorphism and disordered maturation confined to the lower portion of the epidermis. Hyperkeratosis and parakeratosis are present with orthokeratosis at the ostia of appendages leading to the flag or "pink and blue" sign.

Treatment

The inability to predict whether the lesions will persist, regress, or become SCCs makes the management difficult. Treatment is usually advised to avoid any chance of progression to invasive SCC. Treatment modalities for AKs include lesion-targeted therapies such as cryotherapy, curettage, electrosurgery and shave excision and field therapies to treat larger areas of photodamaged skin containing both clinical and subclinical AK lesions approved by US FDA including 5-fluorouracil (5-FU), 5% imiquimod cream, and 3% diclofenac gel. Other options include cryopeeling, dermabrasion, medium and deep chemical peels and photodynamic therapy (PDT).

BASAL CELL CARCINOMA

Non-melanoma skin cancers (NMSCs), specifically basal cell carcinoma (BCC) and squamous cell carcinoma (SCC), represent the most frequently observed malignancy amongst Caucasians. In individuals with fair skin, approximately 75–80% of NMSCs are BCCs and up to 25% are SCCs.

Epidemiology

BCC is more common in elderly individuals, and it usually develops on sun-exposed skin of lighter skinned individuals and is uncommon in dark skin individuals. Men generally have higher rates of BCC than do women (1.5–2:1). Risk factors for BCC include ultraviolet light exposure, northern

European ancestry, light hair and eye color, and inability to tan. Some heritable conditions predispose to the development of multiple BCC such as nevoid basal cell carcinoma syndrome or basal cell nevus syndrome (BCNS), Bazex syndrome and Rombo syndrome.

Clinical Features

BCC typically presents as a shiny, translucent papule or nodule with a smooth surface with arborizing telangiectasias usually present on sun-exposed areas of the head and neck generally the cheeks, forehead, nasolabial folds and eyelids (Fig. 6.5). The tumor enlarges gradually and can ulcerate (rodent ulcer, Fig. 6.6a) and has a characteristic rolled out border.

Features may vary for different clinical subtypes, which include nodular (the most common subtype), morpheaform, superficial (Fig. 6.6b) and fibroepithelioma of Pinkus (FEP). Pigmented BCC is a subtype of nodular BCC seen more commonly in those with darker skin phototypes and exhibits increased melanization (Figs 6.7 and 6.8).

The lesions rarely develop on the palms and soles or mucous membranes and the anatomic location may favor the development of

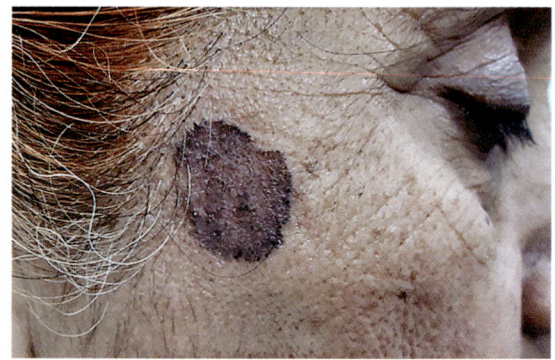

Fig. 6.6b: Superficial BCC

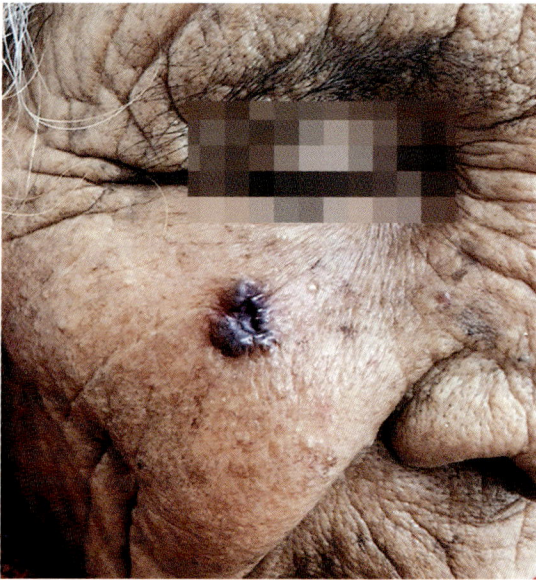

Fig. 6.7: Pigmented basal cell carcinoma: Hyperpigmented papule with rolled out border present over the cheeks in an elderly female

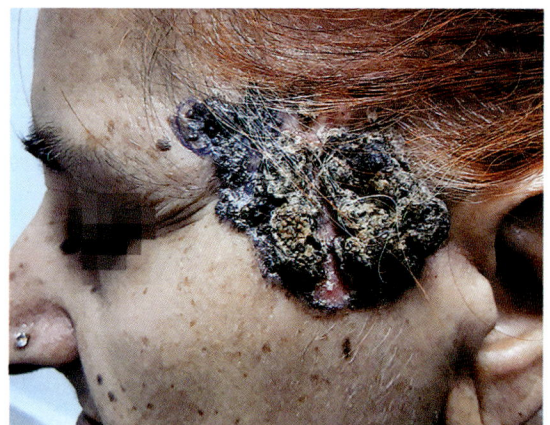

Fig. 6.6a: Ulcerative basal cell carcinoma, also called rodent ulcer. The characteristic border can be appreciated

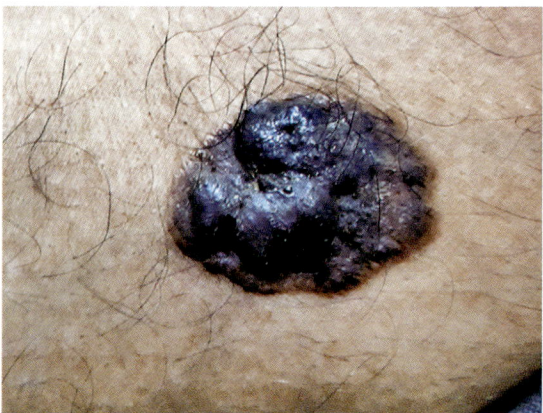

Fig. 6.8: Pigmented basal cell carcinoma

a particular subtype. BCC is a slow-growing tumor that invades locally and rarely metastasizes. Perineural invasion (PNI) is also uncommon and occurs mostly in histologically aggressive or recurrent lesions.

Pathogenesis

The pathogenesis of BCC involves exposure to UV radiation, particularly the UVB spectrum (290–320 nm), that damages DNA and induces mutations in the p53 tumor suppressor gene. It is intense sun exposure rather than prolonged sun exposure that increases the risk of BCC. Other factors involved in the pathogenesis include exposure to ionizing radiation, mutations in regulatory genes and alterations in immunosurveillance.

Pathology

All types of BCC show the presence of aggregations of basaloid keratinocytes within a fibromyxoid stroma. The cells are large with relatively uniform nuclei and scant cytoplasm and the cellular borders are indistinct. A characteristic feature of BCC is retraction of the fibromyxoid stroma around the tumor islands, creating microscopically visible clefts which is useful in differentiating BCCs from other histopathologic simulators.

Treatment

Management of BCC depends on anatomic location and histological features. Approaches include standard surgical excision, Mohs micrographic surgery (MMS), destruction by various modalities such as curettage and desiccation and cryosurgery and topical chemotherapy with 5% imiquimod cream and 5-fluorouracil.

Standard surgical excision with a 4 mm margin is adequate for most cases of non-facial non-morpheaform BCC <2 cm in diameter; however, cure rates are inferior to MMS in the case of recurrent BCC, infiltrative BCC, and BCC arising in high-risk (H) anatomic sites including the embryonic fusion planes.

Radiation therapy is a primary option for treating BCC, if surgery is contraindicated or in cases in which postsurgical margins are positive for cancer.

Recently, hedgehog inhibitors Vismodegib and Sonidegib were approved by the US FDA for the treatment of BCC.

SQUAMOUS CELL CARCINOMA

Cutaneous squamous cell carcinomas (SCCs) are malignant neoplasms arising from suprabasal epidermal keratinocytes. These tumors in most cases develop from precursor lesions of actinic keratosis (AK) and Bowen disease (SCC *in situ*) and represent the second most frequent cutaneous malignancy.

Epidemiology

Majority of SCCs occur in light-skinned individuals older than 60 years, with a male preponderance, on the sun-exposed sites. Other risk factors include ionizing radiation, exposure to environmental carcinogens, immunosuppression, presence of scars and burns, chronic scarring or inflammatory dermatoses, human papillomavirus infection and genodermatoses (xeroderma pigmentosum, albinism).

Clinical Features

The most common presentation of SCC in situ or Bowen's disease (Fig. 6.9) is a slowly enlarging, well-demarcated, erythematous scaly patch or slightly elevated plaque with overlying scale or crust which resembles a psoriatic plaque. Uncommonly, a pigmented variant of BD has been reported.

The lesions are asymptomatic and the development of tenderness, erosion and

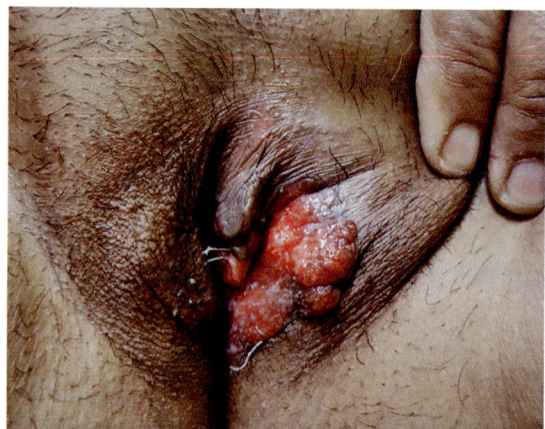

Fig. 6.9: A 50-year-old female presented with non-healing ulcer over labia. Biopsy revealed Bowen's disease

increased diameter may herald evolution into SCC.

Invasive cutaneous SCC presents, usually as a firm, flesh-colored or erythematous, keratotic papule or plaque which may rarely be pigmented, ulcerated verrucous or exophytic (Fig. 6.10a to c). They may be slowly enlarging or rapidly growing and may have significant tenderness and even pain. The head and neck are the most common sites and involvement of legs is seen more commonly in women.

SCCs, like BCC, may cause local tissue destruction, but they also have a significant potential for metastasis generally to regional lymph nodes.

Keratoacanthomas (KAs) are considered to be a variant of SCC and typically present

as rapidly enlarging papules that evolve into crateriform nodules with a central keratotic core over a period of a few weeks (Fig. 6.11). A few authors consider these to represent benign tumors (i.e. pseudomalignancy) since the lesions usually have a tendency of spontaneous regression leaving behind atrophic scars.

Pathogenesis

UV exposure is the predominant cause for non-melanoma skin cancers with cumulative long-term UV exposure rather than intermittent intense episodes of UV exposure increasing the risk for developing SCCs and AKs. The development of SCC from normal keratinocytes begins with UV-induced mutations in the cellular DNA, in particular, p53 gene. This leads to resistance to apoptosis and immune attack, allowing for clonal expansion of the mutated cells and penetration of the basement membrane and invasion into the surrounding tissue.

Pathology

Bowen's disease demonstrates full-thickness atypia in the epidermis including the intra-epidermal portions of the adnexal structures with complete disorganization of the epidermal architecture. Throughout the epidermis, there are numerous atypical, hyperchromatic, pleomorphic keratinocytes showing loss of maturation and polarity and numerous mitotic figures. The hallmark of invasive

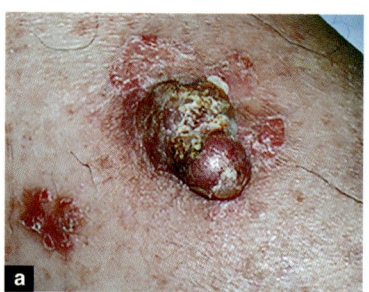
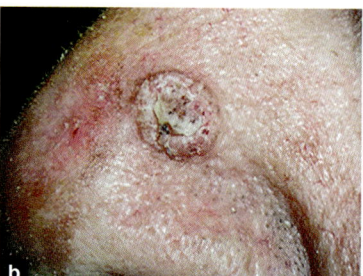
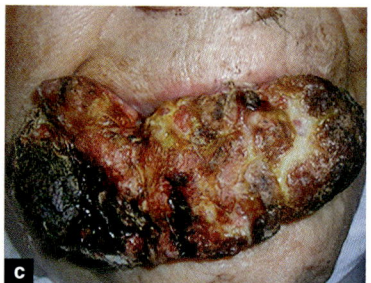

Fig. 6.10: (a) A chronic nodule on the lower leg with ulceration; (b) A nodule with ulceration of the nose; (c) An exophytic tumor of the lower lip

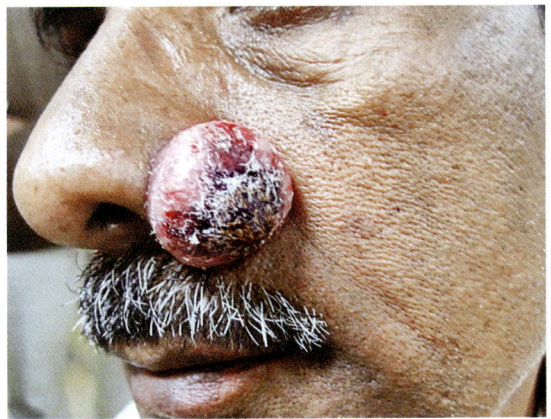

Fig. 6.11: Keratoacanthoma: Rapidly enlarging nodule with a central keratotic core

SCC is the downward extension of atypical keratinocytes beyond the basement membrane and into the dermis.

Treatment

Treatment selection depends on the tumor risk for recurrence and metastasis. Conventional surgical excision is the treatment of choice for small primary SCCs. Recommended margins are 4–6 mm for low-risk lesions and SCCs with a depth of <2 mm; for high-risk lesions with a depth >6 mm or large poorly defined lesions, Mohs micrographic surgery is preferred. Other modalities which can be used alternatively for low-risk lesions are ablative techniques such as electrodesiccation and curettage, liquid nitrogen cryotherapy, carbon dioxide laser, intralesional chemotherapy, and photodynamic therapy.

MELANOCYTIC NEVI

The term 'melanocytic neoplasia' is used to described a heterogeneous group of disorders characterized by the presence of melanocytic cells in epidermal nests or thèque (three or more melanocytic cells in direct contact) within the dermis or other tissues. These neoplasms are referred to as nevi and the cells forming them are called nevomelanocytes.

Nevi are currently subcategorized, based on clinical features and microscopic characteristics, into congenital nevomelanocytic/melanocytic nevi (CNNs), nevus spilus, common acquired nevomelanocytic/melanocytic nevi, blue nevi, pigmented spindle cell nevi (PSCN), Spitz nevi, and nodal nevi.

We will be discussing the common ones that are congenital and acquired melanocytic nevi and Spitz nevi.

Epidemiology

The prevalence of melanocytic nevi is related to age, race, and perhaps genetic and environmental factors. Congenital melanocytic nevi are those that present at birth. Acquired melanocytic nevi can present in early childhood, but their number increases with age, with a peak during the third decade of life; thereafter, they tend to disappear with increasing age. They show equal prevalence in males and females and are more common in those with lighter skin and tend to aggregate in families.

Clinical Features

Acquired melanocytic naevi start as flat, evenly pigmented (junctional) naevi in which melanocytes collect in small groups (nests) along the basal epidermal layer (*see* Fig. 6.12a). As melanocytes migrate down into the dermis, flat moles evolve into raised,

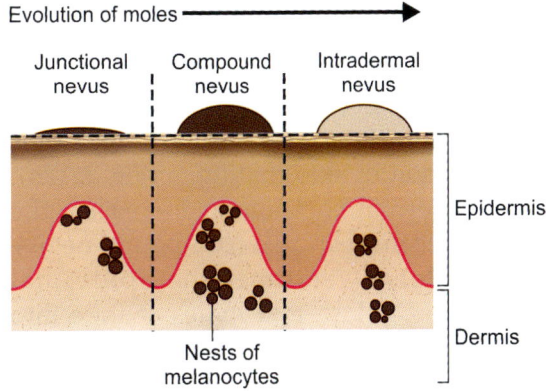

Fig. 6.12a: A depiction of the evolution of moles

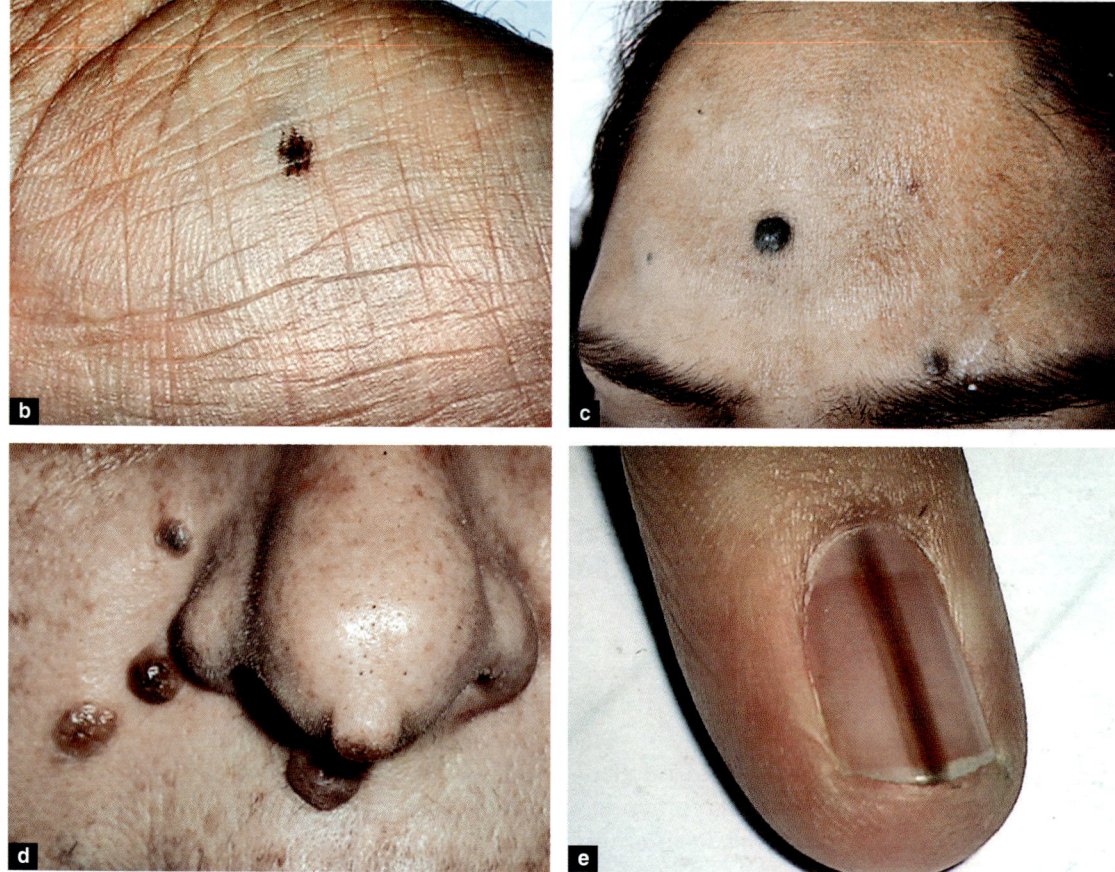

Fig. 6.12b to e: (b) junctional nevus; (c) Compound nevu; (d) Skin-colored dermal nevi; (e) Melanonychia striata due to junctional nevus

lighter or even skin-colored, dome-shaped papules compound dermal melanocytic nevi which may compound hair.

Melanocytic nevi are well-circumscribed, symmetric, round to ovoid lesions, measuring 2 to 6 mm in diameter with regular borders. The junctional nevus is a medium to dark brown macular lesion with slight accentuation of skin markings (Fig. 6.12b). As the dermal component increases, the lesions become elevated (compound nevi—Fig. 6.12c). Over time, the epidermal component is lost, and moles change into flesh-colored or pale brown papules (intradermal melanocytic naevi—Fig. 6.12d), before disappearing in old age. Junctional

activity can lead to black bands of the nail (Fig. 6.12e).

A new pigmented growth in an elderly patient is much more likely to be a seborrheic wart, solar lentigo, or melanoma than a melanocytic nevus.

Congenital melanocytic nevi are on average larger than acquired nevi and classified as small (<1.5 cm in greatest diameter), intermediate- or medium-sized (1.5 to 19.9 cm), and large or giant (>20 cm). The lesions are usually smooth, regular, sharply demarcated and slightly raised at birth and hypertrichosis may be present (Fig. 6.13). As a child grows, the CNN grows relatively proportionally and continues to

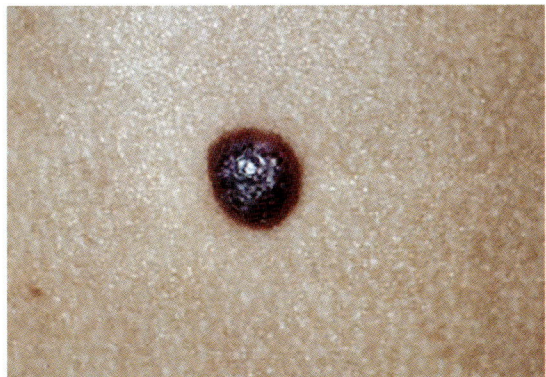

Fig. 6.13: Spitz nevus presenting as a solitary dome-shaped, hyperpigmented nodule

mature, i.e. color darkening and the surface may become more elevated and verrucous. CNNs of the head, neck, or posterior midline and large CNN with associated multiple satellite lesions may be complicated by underlying cranial or spinal leptomeningeal melanocytosis. Sudden appearance of a dermal or subcutaneous nodule, itching, pain, bleeding, or ulceration may indicate malignant degeneration which is more common in larger lesions.

Pathogenesis

Environmental exposure to UVR appears to be a critical inciting or permissive factor for the development of melanocytic nevi. Melanocytic nevi result from the proliferation of slightly altered melanocytic stem cells present in the epidermis, which when needed to replenish melanocytes produce nevomelanocytes or nevus cells instead. When these nevus cells are present in the epidermis, they form junctional nevi. Subsequently, migration into the dermis gives rise to compound nevi and ultimately dermal nevi when no residual nevus cells are present within the epidermis.

Pathology

Melanocytic nevi contain intraepidermal and/or dermal collections of nevus cells

arranged in nests separated from epidermis by a retraction artifact. In contrast to acquired nevi that are confined to the papillary and upper reticular dermis, CNN may show infiltration of the lower reticular dermis, subcutaneous fat and even deeper.

Treatment

Majority of acquired nevomelanocytic nevi require no treatment. Indications for removing melanocytic nevi include cosmetic concern, repeated irritation and atypical clinical appearance suspicious for melanoma. Complete removal of nevi is best accomplished by excision. Destructive modes of therapy (electrodesiccation, dermabrasion and laser) should be avoided as leaving a partially excised nevus can lead to repigmentation and regrowth (pseudomelanoma).

The treatment of CNN depends on the risk of melanoma and cosmetic concerns or anatomic location and presence of neuro-cutaneous melanosis. The routine excision of uniform-appearing small and medium congenital nevi is not advised due to the low melanoma risk. Since melanoma may arise in large CNNs even in the first year of life, excision should be considered as early as possible usually after the first 6 months of age to reduce surgical risks. The treatment goal is the removal of the nevus while preserving function and improving cosmetic appearance. Extensive involvement may necessitate abandoning prophylactic excision and accepting lifelong surveillance to detect the earliest signs of malignant change.

PIGMENTED SPINDLE CELL NEVUS (PIGMENTED SPITZ NEVUS)

As with other melanocytic nevi, pigmented spindle cell nevi are derived from nevus cells but have prominent spindle cell features. They present as homogeneous, dark brown

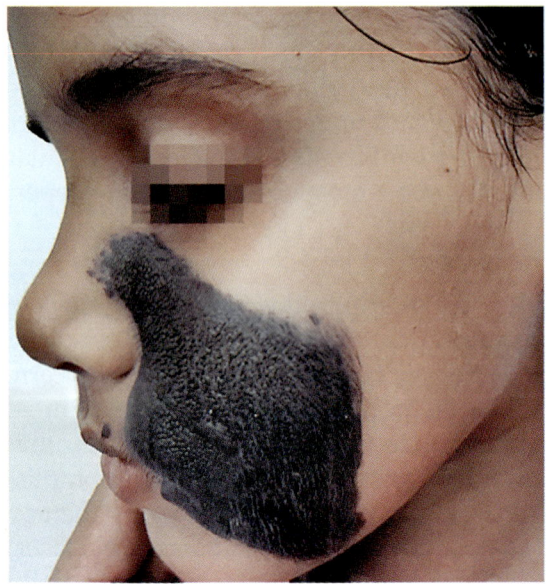

Fig. 6.14: An intermediate-sized congenital melanocytic nevus in a 6-year-old girl. Note the hair growth on the lesion

to black flat or slightly raised, well-circumscribed lesion, usually <6 mm in diameter found in children or young adults since 6 months (Fig. 6.14).

Although atypical variants have been described, transformation to cutaneous melanoma is rare. Histopathologic examination is generally required for diagnosis of pigmented spindle cell nevi. The treatment of pigmented spindle cell nevi is complete excision with clear margins.

ATYPICAL (DYSPLASTIC) MELANOCYTIC NEVUS

These nevi are flat (totally or partially with central elevation), large (>5 mm) lesions with irregular shape, variable pigmentation and indistinct borders present most frequently on sun-exposed areas, especially intermittently exposed like the back. These lesions occur in a familial pattern and most lesions are associated with large numbers of common acquired nevi. Though majority of lesions involute and disappear over time,

atypical nevi are markers for risk of melanoma. Histologic features include an immature disordered growth pattern with random cytologic atypia in melanocytes and a lymphocytic host response. The treatment for atypical nevi is observation and careful follow-up to look for malignant transformation.

MELANOMA

Melanoma represents a malignant tumor arising from melanocytes, leading to >75% of skin cancer deaths due to its metastatic potential.

Epidemiology

The incidence of melanoma has significantly increased worldwide over the last a few decades. It develops almost exclusively in light-skinned populations with a mean age of diagnosis at 52 years. The incidence rises with age, especially in men after the age of 40.

Clinical Features

The well-known acronym for melanoma detection is ABCD; A stands for asymmetry, B for border (irregular poorly defined borders), C for color (having varying shades) and D for diameter (i.e. greater than 6 mm). Another diagnostic aid is the "ugly duckling" sign where a pigmented lesion different from other pigmented lesions in an individual should be approached with a high index of suspicion. Cutaneous melanomas present with variable manifestations and are classified into subtypes based on clinical features and histologic findings.

Superficial spreading melanoma (SSM) is the most common type most frequently seen on the trunk in men and legs in women (Fig. 6.15a). It arises either *de novo* or in a pre-existing nevus. The melanoma starts as a macule showing a slow horizontal (radial)

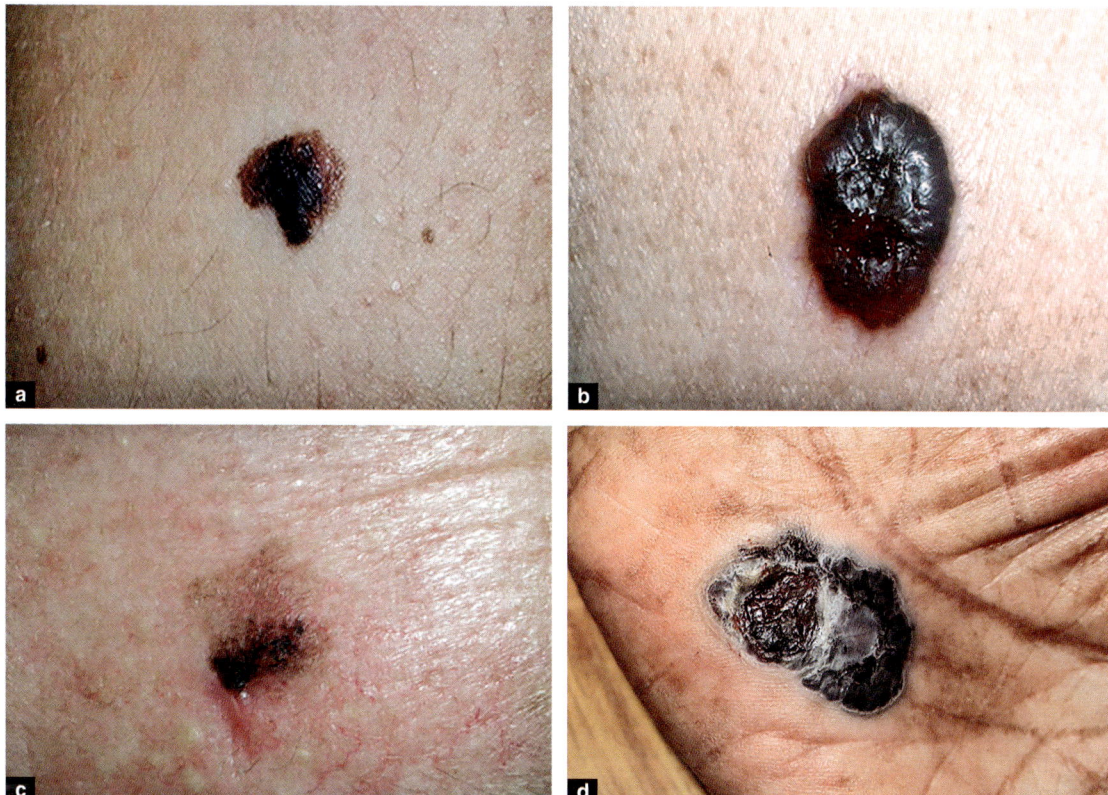

Fig. 6.15a to d: (a) Supercial spreading melanoma *in situ*; (b) Nodular malignant melanoma; (c) Lentigo maligna presenting as a hyperpigmented lesion with irregular borders located on the forehead; (d) Acral lentiginous melanoma in a 45-year-old male (*Courtesy:* Dr Ananta Khurana)

growth phase when in situ and development of a papule or nodule correlates with a more rapid vertically oriented growth phase.

Nodular melanoma is the second most common type presenting as a blue to black nodule which may be ulcerated or bleeding developing rapidly over several weeks to months (Fig. 6.15b). They usually begin *de novo* than arising in a pre-existing nevus and do not have a horizontal growth phase. The trunk is the most common site. Early lesions often lack asymmetry and have regular borders and a few lesions are amelanotic.

Lentigo maligna melanoma (*LMM*) represents a minority of cutaneous melanomas occurring in chronically sun-damaged skin, most commonly on the face, the nose and cheek in particular, during the seventh decade of life. They arise in a precursor lesion termed lentigo maligna (*in situ* melanoma) (Fig. 6.15c).

Acral lentiginous melanoma (*ALM*) is the most common form in darker-pigmented individuals. The most common site for ALM is the palm (Fig. 6.15d) and soles followed by in and around the nail apparatus. Melanoma of the nail matrix can present as widening, dark, or irregularly pigmented longitudinal melanonychia or as pigmentation extending onto the hyponychium or the proximal nail fold (Hutchinson sign).

Pathogenesis

Both genetic and environmental factors play a role in melanoma pathogenesis. Periodic, intense ultraviolet (UV) exposure during childhood and adolescence, is a major environmental cause of melanoma. Other risk factors include light skin pigmentation, blond or red hair, blue eyes, Fitzpatrick skin phototype I-II, presence of associated melanocytic nevi (increased numbers and atypical nevi lesions), positive family history, history of prior melanoma, mutation in p16, BRAF, or MC1R and xeroderma pigmentosum.

The critical step in tumor progression of melanoma is the transition from radial to vertical growth phases with a property of aggregative growth which finally leads to metastatic malignant melanoma.

Pathology

The gold standard for diagnosing melanoma is histopathologic evaluation. The histologic diagnosis of melanoma is based on architectural and cytologic features. The presence of cytologic atypia, referring to cellular and nuclear enlargement, nuclear pleomorphism and hyperchromasia, nucleolar variability and the presence of mitoses in the deep dermis is essential to diagnose melanoma. The architectural features consistent with melanoma include asymmetry, poor circumscription, large size (>5–6 mm) and variability in the size and shape of nests of melanocytes in the lower epidermis and dermis with tendency to become confluent and lack of maturation with descent into the dermis. Immunohistochemical staining for melanocyte differentiation antigens, namely gp100 (HMB45), tyrosinase and Melan-A/MART-1 may be useful for the diagnosis of melanoma, in poorly differentiated neoplasms containing little or no pigment.

Treatment

The standard of therapy for primary cutaneous melanoma is wide local excision with histopathologically confirmed tumor-free margins to prevent local recurrence due to persistent disease. Current recommended clinical margins for melanoma *in situ* and lentigo maligna is 0.5 cm, for melanoma with a <1 mm Breslow depth is 1 cm, for melanoma 1–2 mm thick is 1–2 cm as possible, and for melanoma >2 mm thick is 2 cm. For microscopic or macroscopic involvement of lymph nodes, complete lymph node dissection should be done. High-dose interferon-α 2b (IFN-α 2b) is the adjuvant therapy approved by the US FDA post-surgery for patients at high risk for relapse, such as, primary melanoma >4 mm with ulceration or presence of nodal disease.

Bibliography

1. Bolognia JL, Jorizzo JJ. Schaffer JV. Dermatology. 3rd ed. London: Elsevier. 2012. Chapter 108 Actinic Keratosis, Basal Cell Carcinoma and Squamous Cell Carcinoma; p. 1773–94.

2. Bolognia JL, Jorizzo JJ. Schaffer JV. Dermatology. 3rd ed. London: Elsevier. 2012. Chapter 109 Benign Epidermal Tumors and Proliferations; p. 1795–1816.

3. Bolognia JL, Jorizzo JJ. Schaffer JV. Dermatology. 3rd ed. London: Elsevier. 2012. Chapter 113 Melanoma; p. 1885–1914.

4. Goldsmith LA, Katz SI, Gilchrest BA, Paller AS, Leffell DA, Wolff K. Fitzpatrick's Dermatology In General Medicine. 8th ed. New York : McGraw-Hill Medical, 2012. Chapter 113. Epithelial precancerous lesions. p1261–82.

5. Goldsmith LA, Katz SI, Gilchrest BA, Paller AS, Leffell DA, Wolff K. Fitzpatrick's Dermatology In General Medicine. 8th ed. New York : McGraw-Hill Medical, 2012. Chapter 114. Squamous Cell Carcinoma p1283–93.

6. Goldsmith LA, Katz SI, Gilchrest BA, Paller AS, Leffell DA, Wolff K. Fitzpatrick's Dermatology In General Medicine. 8th ed. New York : McGraw-Hill Medical, 2012. Chapter 115. Basal Cell Carcinoma. p1294–1303.

7. Goldsmith LA, Katz SI, Gilchrest BA, Paller AS, Leffell DA, Wolff K. Fitzpatrick's Dermatology In General Medicine. 8th ed. New York : McGraw-Hill Medical, 2012. Section 22. Melanocytic tumours . p1377–1444.

8. National Comprehensive Cancer Network. Basal cell cancer (Version 1.2018). https://www.nccn.org/professionals/physician_gls/pdf/nmsc.pdf Accessed February 6, 2018.

9. National Comprehensive Cancer Network. Melanoma (Version 2.2018 https://www.nccn.org/professionals/physician_gls/pdf/melanoma.pdf Accessed February 6, 2018.

10. National Comprehensive Cancer Network. Squamous cell skin cancer (Version 2.2018). https://www.nccn.org/professionals/physician_gls/pdf/squamous.pdf Accessed February 6, 2018.

Treatment Options for Hyperpigmentation

Gauri Vats

Disorders of hyperpigmentation can be inherited or acquired, resulting from alterations occurring at any level in the melanogenesis pathway. The understanding of pigment formation and of the pathogenetic mechanisms underlying these disorders is important for targeting the correct pigmentation pathway. In this chapter, we have given an overview of the skin lightening agents available for these disorders.

TOPICAL SKIN-LIGHTENING AGENTS

Depigmentation formulations contain one or several different active compounds that can be classified according to their mechanism of action (Fig. 7.1). Here, we have classified them according to their structure as phenolic and non-phenolic compounds. Table 7.1 depicts the agents with their mechanism of action.

Phenolic Compounds

Hydroquinone

Hydroquinone remains the most prescribed bleaching agent worldwide, and is still the gold standard for treatment of hyperpigmentation. Being structurally similar to melanin precursors, it acts by inhibiting tyrosinase, reduces DNA and RNA synthesis and

Table 7.1: Mode of action of skin-lightening agents

Mechanism of action	Depigmenting agent
Tyrosinase inhibition	Hydroquinone, mequinol, arbutin, kojic acid, azelaic acid, licorice
Stimulation of epidermal turnover	Retinoids
Interaction with copper	Kojic acid, ascorbic acid
Inhibition of melanosome maturation	Arbutin, deoxyarbutin
Reduction in melanosome transfer	Retinoids, soy
Inhibition of plasmin	Tranexamic acid

enhances melanosome degradation with melanocyte destruction. It is considered to be pregnancy category C drug. The concentrations employed usually vary from 2 to 5%. It is normally applied once a day and results are appreciable after 4 to 6 weeks, whereas optimal effects are observed after 6 to 10 weeks of treatment.

Hydroquinone has been combined with many other agents to exploit the synergistic action of each compound in a mixture. Kligman and Willis, in 1975, performed an early study assessing the clinical efficacy of

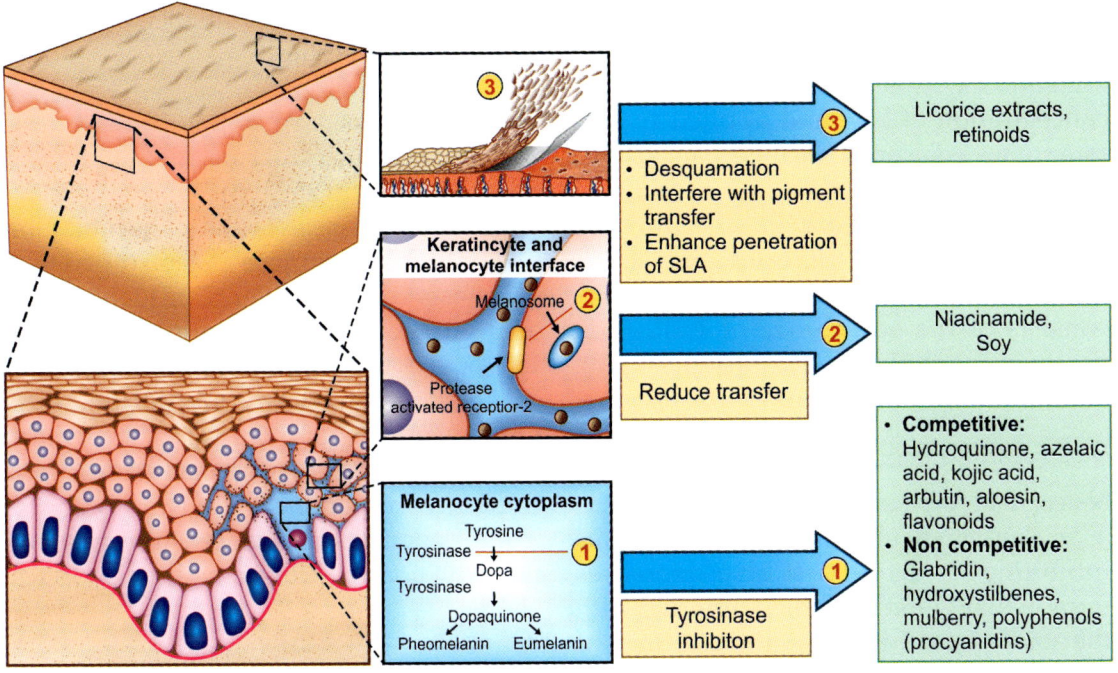

Fig. 7.1: Mechanism of action of common agents (SLA: Skin lightening agent)

hydroquinone. The Kligman formulation, comprised of 5% hydroquinone with 0.1% tretinoin and 0.1% dexamethasone, was the earliest combination. Tretinoin facilitates the removal of pigment by accelerating the keratinocytes' turnover, enhances hydroquinone penetration through the stratum corneum, and protects hydroquinone from oxidation. The corticosteroid is aimed to reduce inflammation as a side effect of both hydroquinone and tretinoin, but it also inhibits melanocyte metabolism. Long-term use of this preparation may result in skin atrophy, telangiectasia, erythema, rosacea-like acneiform eruptions, increased growth of vellus hair, and perioral dermatitis. The US Food and Drug Administration (FDA) has approved a modified combination of the Kligman formulation, containing 4% hydroquinone, 0.05% tretinoin, and 0.01% fluocinolone acetonide.

Side effects induced by hydroquinone include infrequent allergic reactions, post-inflammatory hyperpigmentation, and transient hypochromia. Chronic adverse events consist of leukomelanoderma en confetti, exogenous ochronosis, and nail discoloration. Exogenous ochronosis is a rare side effect consisting of a blue-black pigmentation of the treated areas. It tends to resolve slowly after stopping the application. Exposure to sunlight causes repigmentation in patients using hydroquinone which can be prevented by using broad-spectrum sunscreen.

Permanent bleaching of skin and ochronosis are the most dreadful consequences which led to its withdrawal. Many authors have focused on the potential mutagenicity.

Monobenzone

It is the monobenzyl ether of hydroquinone, that has an indication confined to the achievement of a permanent depigmentation of normal skin surrounding vitiliginous areas. It acts by permanently damaging the melanocytes through the release of reactive free radicals produced by tyrosine-mediated metabolism. It is usually prepared at a concentration of 20% and applied two or three times a day on pigmented skin. Results are appreciable after 6 to 12 months of treatment. Side effects include burning sensation after use, satellite depigmentation in distant sites, and "consort vitiligo," which consists of the occurrence of vitiligo in persons cohabiting with patients using monobenzone.

N-acetyl-4-S-cysteaminylphenol

N-acetyl-4-S-cysteaminylphenol (NCAP) acts as an alternative substrate of tyrosinase, thus inhibiting its activity. It also decreases intracellular glutathione by interfering with the thiol system, favoring the pathway of pheomelanin. Compared to hydroquinone, it seems to be more stable and less irritating.

Hydroquinone Monomethyl Ether (4-Hydroxyanisole, Mequinol)

Another derivative of hydroquinone, it is oxidized inside melanocytes, leading to the formation of cytotoxic quinones. The bleaching effect is consequent to the destruction of melanocytes.

Non-Phenolic Compounds

Arbutin and Deoxyarbutin

Arbutin is a natural β-D-glucopyranoside derivative of hydroquinone, extracted from Uva-ursi folium (bearberry plant). Compared to hydroquinone, it seems to be less cytotoxic. Arbutin's mechanism of action is based on the inhibition of both tyrosinase and 5, 6-dihydroxyindole-2-carboxylic acid (DHICA) polymerase and inhibition of melanosome maturation without associated melanocyte toxicity. Higher concentration may provide additional therapeutic benefit but paradoxic darkening may occur. Deoxyarbutin, a modified synthetic derivative of arbutin, has been developed with enhanced pigment lightening properties.

Azelaic Acid

The lightening effect of azelaic acid, a naturally occurring dicarboxylic acid derived from P. ovale, is due to the inhibition not only of tyrosinase but also of DNA synthesis and of several mitochondrial oxido-reductases. It is commonly used at 15% or 20% concentration for the treatment of acne and hyperpigmentation. It is pregnancy category B drug. Mild irritant contact dermatitis is the main side effect. Unlike hydroquinone, it targets only abnormal melanocytes and hence will not lighten skin with normally functioning melanocytes.

Kojic Acid

Kojic acid is a hydrophilic fungal metabolite produced by Aspergillus spp and Penicillium spp. Its mechanism of action is based on the ability to chelate copper, which inactivates tyrosinase and suppresses the tautomerization from dopachrome to DHICA. Formulations used are 0.75–1%, 2%, 4% in cream base. It is used alone or in combination with tretinoin, hydroquinone and acts synergistically with glycolic acid. It is unstable in cosmetic formulation and on exposure to sunlight or air, it loses its efficacy. Kojic dipalmitate is a more stable alternative. Main adverse effects are mild facial erythema, high potential for causing sensitization and irritant dermatitis.

Licorice

Derived from the roots of Glycyrrhiza glabra, glabridin is the hydrophobic fraction of liquorice. It has dual pigment modulating and anti-inflammatory properties. Active ingredients are flavonoids, liquirtin and isoliquirtin. It prevents UVB-induced pigmentation and also inhibits tyrosinase, cyclo-oxygenase activity and superoxide anion production. Bleaching activity of liquiritin is related to its ability to disperse melanin and to remove melanodermic and epidermal stain. Licorice extract is considered a weak lightening agent and must be combined with other agents for optimal clinical results.

Flavonoid-like Agents

Flavonoids are natural polyphenolic compounds with well-known anti-inflammatory, antioxidant, antiviral and anticarcinogenic properties. Among flavonoids, oxyresveratrol, catechin conjugated to gallic acid, ellagic acid and aloesin have hypopigmenting effects.

Catechin and gallic acid derive from green tea leaves. Ellagic acid naturally occurs in a variety of plants, such as strawberry, green tea, eucalyptus and geranium. It prevents UV-induced pigmentation and inhibits dose-dependent and noncompetitive tyrosinase by chelating copper at the active site of the enzyme.

Aloesin, isolated from the aloe plant, acts as a competitive inhibitor of tyrosinase, inhibiting both hydroxylation of tyrosine to dihydroxyphenylalanine (DOPA) and oxidation of DOPA to dopaquinone. Recent studies have highlighted that its bleaching ability is greater than that of arbutin and kojic acid. Furthermore, aloesin is non-mutagenic.

Alpha-Hydroxy Acids

Alpha-hydroxy acids like glycolic acid and lactic acid can also be used for the treatment of hyperpigmentation. They act by influencing cellular epidermal turnover, cause pigment dispersion, and inhibit tyrosinase activity.

Ascorbic Acid

Affects melanogenesis by reducing o-dopaquinone to DOPA thus acting as an antioxidant and quenching free radicals caused by the absorption of UV radiation. Being highly unstable, it oxidizes and easily decomposes in aqueous solution. Some ascorbate esters have been developed which obviate these effects.

Retinoids

Retinoids affect multiple steps of the melanization pathway. They cause rapid epidermal turnover, hence increasing the dispersion of melanin granules.

In lighter skin types, retinoid treatment stimulates tyrosinase activity, whereas such activity does not occur in dark complexions. It has been suggested that this effect is mediated by keratinocytes derived cytokines that incite melanin production in melanocytes with a low constitutive level of melanogenesis.

Soybean

Exerts its effect via inhibition of the protease-activated receptor-2 (PAR-2), on keratinocytes, that plays an important role in the modulation of melanosomes' phagocytosis.

Niacinamide

It is the biologically active amide of vitamin B_3, effects being anti-inflammatory, antioxidant and immunomodulatory. It reduces melanosome transfer by interfering with the interaction between keratinocytes and melanocytes. Niacinamide is a popular ingredient of many cosmeceutical creams available in the Indian market as shown in Table 7.2.

Conclusion

It is important to note that since melanin is a key natural skin protectant, the aim of depigmenting therapies is mostly to even skin tone and bleach only hyperpigmented areas, without affecting the inherent skin color. All formulations should include or be

Table 7.2: Major ingredients of various cosmeceutical creams available in the Indian market

Preparation	Active ingredient
Fair and Lovely	Niacinamide
Clean and Clear	Niacinamide, fruit extract
Ponds White	Niacinamide, allantoin, vitamin E, fatty acids
Lakme	Niacinamide, allantoin, vitamin E
Olay	Niacinamide, vitamin E, fatty acids
Garnier	Vitamin C, fruit extract, sugarcane extract, lemon extract
Patanjali	Aloe vera, mulethi, oils

accompanied by the daily use of a high SPF sunscreen. Plant extracts/botanical extracts are becoming popular nowadays due to their excellent safety profile and are being widely used for epidermal hyperpigmentation. Through careful choice of the ingredient, the clinician can confidently determine the best course for the individual patient.

Bibliography

1. Hakozaki T, Minwalla L, Zhuang J, et al. The effect of niacinamide on reducing cutaneous pigmentation and suppression of melanosome transfer. Br J Dermatol 2002;147:20–31.
2. Halder RM, Richards GM. Management of dyschromias in ethnic skin. Dermatol Ther 2004; 17:151–7.
3. Jones K, Hughes J, Hong M, et al. Modulation of melanogenesis by aloesin: a competitive inhibitor of tyrosinase. Pigment Cell Res 2002;15:335–40.
4. Kligman AM, Willis I. A new formula for depigmenting human skin. Arch Dermatol 1975;111:40–8.
5. Kooyers TJ, Westerhof W. Toxicology and health risks of hydroquinone in skin lightening formulations. J Eur Acad Dermatol Venereol 2006;20: 777–80.
6. Nordlund JJ, Grimes PE, Ortonne JPJ. The safety of hydroquinone. J Eur Acad Dermatol Venereol 2006;20:781–7.
7. Seiberg M, Paine C, Sharlow E, et al. Inhibition of melanosome transfer results in skin lightening. J Invest Dermatol 2000;115:162–7.
8. Usuki A, Ohashi A, Sato H, et al. The inhibitory effect of glycolic acid and lactic acid on melanin synthesis in melanoma cells. Exp Dermatol 2003; 2(Suppl 12):43–50.
9. Zawar VP, Mhaskar ST. Exogenous ochronosis following hydroquinone for melasma. J Cosmet Dermatol 2004;3:234–6.

Phototherapy

Niharika Dixit, Manu Sehrawat

PHOTOTHERAPY IN VITILIGO

Phototherapy is the most commonly used treatment modality in extensive vitiligo (Fig. 8.1). Different forms of phototherapy for vitiligo include broadband UVB (BB-UVB), narrowband-UVB (NB-UVB), excimer light and excimer laser, and psoralen plus UVA (PUVA). The roots of phototherapy in vitiligo can be traced to before 1500 BC when Indians used extracts from the plants *Ammi majus* and *Psoralen corylifolia* and sunlight for treating "leukoderma". A similar form of heliotherapy was performed in ancient Egypt. In 1947, these plants were found by Fahmy et al. to contain 8-methoxypsoralen (8-MOP) and 5-MOP. Since the middle of the last century, PUVA or photo chemotherapy had been the most popular form of phototherapy for patients with vitiligo. However, in recent years, it has been gradually superseded by NB-UVB, which has been shown by various studies to have greater efficacy and fewer adverse effects than PUVA. This was first reported by Westerhof and Nieuweboer-Krobotova in 1997.

In India though the simplest form of phototherapy is PUVA-sol which utilizes the abundant sunlight.

Mechanism of Action and Rationale for the Treatment

In vitiligo, there is a complete or subtotal loss of melanocytes in the lesional skin. Melanocytes in the bulb and infundibulum of the hair follicle are destroyed in vitiliginous skin, whereas inactive cells in the middle and lower parts of the follicle and the outer root sheath are spared.

NB-UVB

The immunomodulatory effects of NB-UVB are important for repigmentation in active vitiligo. It stimulates epidermal expression of interleukin-10, which induces differentiation of T-regulatory lymphocytes which inhibits the activity of autoreactive T lymphocytes. UV radiation promotes the proliferation and migration of melanocytes located in the perilesional skin, and enhances activation of immature melanocytes in the outer root sheath of hair follicles. This process is known as "biostimulation" and this is the major repigmenting mechanism of NB-UVB in stable vitiligo.

NB-UVB irradiation increases the expression of endothelin-1 and basic fibroblast growth factor by keratinocytes,

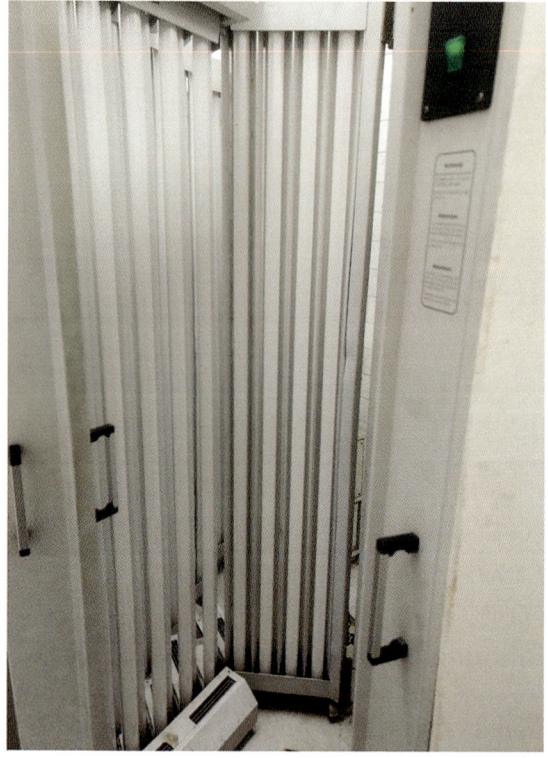

Fig. 8.1: Phototherapy unit

which in turn may promote melanocyte proliferation. In addition to this, it also induces phosphorylated focal adhesion kinase (FAK) expression and matrix metalloproteinase (MMP)-2 activity in melanocytes, leading to increased melanocyte migration. UVB irradiation has long been known to increase human skin pigmentation through enhancement of the number of DOPA-positive melanocytes, synthesis of melanin by melanocytes, and transfer of melanin from melanocytes to keratinocytes. More recently, an increase in human melanocyte DNA synthesis has been demonstrated following UVB radiation exposure.

PUVA

Following activation by light, methoxsalen (photosensitizer) forms covalent bonds with DNA, resulting in the generation of single-stranded and double-stranded DNA adducts. PUVA phototherapy has also been found to stimulate the release of melanocyte growth factors by keratinocytes, induce proliferation of melanocytes, enhance melanocyte migration (by inducing MMP-2 secretion), stimulate melanogenesis, and decrease the expression of vitiligo-associated antigens on melanocyte cell membranes. In addition, treatment with PUVA may induce lymphocyte apoptosis, and induces differentiation of T-regulatory lymphocytes with suppressor activity.

Excimer Laser and Excimer Light

It has similar actions as that of NB-UVB.

TREATMENT PROTOCOLS

Whole body phototherapy is the main treatment option available for the treatment of generalized non-segmental vitiligo with over 15–20% body surface area involvement. For localized vitiligo, targeted phototherapy allows for selective treatment of lesional skin, thus avoiding side effects in unaffected areas, and allowing higher doses to be achieved as well as larger dose increments. Different targeted devices have been introduced and studied, including 308 nm excimer laser, monochromatic excimer light (MEL) and several broadband UVA- and UVB-targeted light sources.

NB-UVB

It is characterized by polychromatic light with a peak emission wavelength of 311 to 313 nm. Phototherapy protocol consists of exposure to ultraviolet radiation (UVR) two to three times a week (earlier repigmentation makes thrice weekly dosing optimal). There are two dosing protocols—based on minimal erythema dose (MED) and based on Fitzpatrick's skin type (Table 8.1). The Vitiligo Working Group recommends

Table 8.1: Dosing guidelines for narrowband-UVB (NB-UVB)

1. According to MED

Initial UVB	50%
Treatments 1–20	Increased by 10% of MED
Treatments ≥21	Increased by 20% of MED

MED determination

Expose 1 cm² areas on lower back or inner aspect of forearm

Skin type						
I, II	100	200	300	400	500	600
III, IV	200	400	600	800	1000	1200
V	400	600	800	1000	1200	1400

*If skin type VI, use a skin type based regime

2. According to skin type

Skin type	Initial UVB dose, mJ/cm²	Maximum dose, mJ/cm²
I	130	2000
II	220	2000
III	260	3000
IV	330	3000
V	350	5000
VI	400	5000

initiation with 200 mJ/cm² regardless of constitutive skin type and increase by 10–20% per treatment. Repigmentation is expected during the first 48 treatments (in case of slow responders > 72 exposures). The face and neck are the most responsive sites to phototherapy, which are areas with large number of hair follicles, whereas acral sites, nipples and lips are the least responsive. Once maximal response is obtained, phototherapy is usually tapered and discontinued (Table 8.2).

Broadband UVB (BB-UVB)

BB-UVB (290 to 320 nm), originally used for psoriasis, particularly in combination with coal tar by William Goeckerman, has been used in various diseases including vitiligo. Very few reports have shown repigmentation with BB-UVB, also with the development of NB-UVB, use of BB-UVB in vitiligo is obsolete.

PUVA

It has been the mainstay therapy for generalized vitiligo since 1951 until it got replaced by NB-UVB. In this, the patient first ingests a photosensitizer (8-methoxypsoralen: 0.4–0.6 mg/kg) or apply methoxsalen in solution or cream form (in localized vitiligo), and then after 120 minutes (20–30 minutes in case of topical) patient is exposed to UVA (320–400 nm) irradiation. The dosing regimes are given in Table 8.3.

Broadband Ultraviolet A

Only one study has shown its effectiveness in vitiligo. Therefore, it is rarely used.

Visible Light

Visible light, in the form of low energy helium-neon laser (wavelength 632.8 nm), has been shown to be effective for segmental vitiligo, particularly in children with

Table 8.2: The vitiligo working group (VWG) phototherapy consensus recommendations

Frequency of administration
- Optimal: 3 times per week
- Acceptable: 2 times per week

Dosing protocol
- Initiate dose at 200 mJ/cm^2 irrespective of skin type
- Increase by 10 to 20% per treatment
- Fixed dosing based on skin type is another acceptable dosing strategy that takes inherent differences in the minimal erythema dose (MED) of various skin types into account

Maximum acceptable dose
- Face: 1500 mJ/cm^2
- Body: 3000 mJ/cm^2

Maximum number of exposures
- Skin phototype IV–VI: No limit
- Skin phototype I–III: More data on the risk of cutaneous malignancy is needed before a recommendation can be made

Course of narrowband ultraviolet B (NB-UVB)
- Assess treatment response after 18 to 36 exposures
- Minimum number of doses needed to determine lack of response: 48 exposures
- Due to the existence of slow responders, up to 72 exposures may be needed to determine lack of response to phototherapy

Dose adjustment based on degree of erythema
- No erythema: Increase next dose by 10 to 20%
- Pink asymptomatic erythema: Hold at current dose until erythema disappears then increase by 10 to 20%
- Bright red asymptomatic erythema: Stop phototherapy until affected areas become light pink, then resume at last tolerated dose
- Symptomatic erythema (includes pain and blistering): Stop phototherapy until the skin heals and erythema fades to a light pink, then resume at last tolerated dose

Dose adjustment following missed doses
- 4 to 7 days between treatments: Hold dose constant
- 8 to 14 days between treatments: Decrease dose by 25%
- 15 to 21 days between treatments: Decrease dose by 50%
- More than 3 weeks between treatments: Re-start at initial dose

Tapering NB-UVB after complete repigmentation achieved
- First month: Phototherapy twice weekly
- Second month: Phototherapy once weekly
- Third and fourth months: Phototherapy every other week
- After 4 months: Discontinue phototherapy

Follow-up
- Skin phototype I–III: Yearly follow-up for total body skin examination to monitor for adverse effects of phototherapy, including cutaneous malignancy
- Skin phototype IV–VI: No need to return for safety monitoring, as no reports of malignancy exist with this group
- All patients: Return on relapse for treatment

Table 8.3: Dosing guidelines for PUVA

1. *MPD* (*minimum phototoxic dose*) *based*

- MPD Determination-expose 1 cm² areas on lower back or inner aspect of forearm to 0.5, 1.0, 2.0, 3.0, 4.0, 5.0 mJ/cm²-read after 72 hours
- Initial exposure: 50–70% of MPD
- Subsequent exposure: 2–4 times per week

2. According to skin type

Skin type	Initial UVA dose, mJ/cm²	Increment per week, mJ/cm²
I	0.5	0.5
II	1.0	0.5
III	1.5	0.5
IV	2.0	0.5
V	2.5	0.5
VI	3.0	0.5

periorbital and perioral lesions. The mechanism being increased melanocyte proliferation, differentiation and migration along with increased microcirculation.

6. Targeted Phototherapy

Targeted phototherapy also known as focused phototherapy, concentrated or microphototherapy, delivers therapeutic doses of UVR only to lesional skin, unlike the above mentioned techniques which expose both involved and uninvolved skin to UVR. These devices offer many advantages over conventional phototherapy:

- These can be used on treatment resistant lesions.
- Exposure of involved areas only and sparing of uninvolved areas, thus minimizing acute side effects such as erythema and long-term risk of skin cancer on unaffected skin.
- Short duration of treatment—less frequent visits.
- Delivery of higher doses (supererythemogenic doses) of energy selectively to the lesions thereby enhancing efficacy and achieving faster response.
- The maneuvrable handpiece allows treatment of difficult areas such as the scalp, nose, genitals, oral mucosa and ear.
- Easy administration for children as delivery is handheld.
- Machines occupy less space.

The limitations of targeted phototherapy include expensive machines and not suitable for patients with more than 10% involvement.

Excimer Laser

The excimer laser is characterized by a wavelength of 308 nm (similar to NB-UVB), and is generated using xenon and chlorine gases. It emits a monochromatic wavelength at high irradiance (defined as power output per unit area). This allows the selective treatment of the lesional skin, also the perilesional skin remain unaffected. Treatment is started with a low dose of 100 mJ/cm² subsequently increased by 10–20% depending on the erythema. Doses are given twice weekly.

Monochromatic Excimer Light/ Excimer Lamp (MEL)

The monochromatic excimer light (excimer lamp), like excimer laser, also emits light with 308 nm wavelength. It has also been shown to be equally effective in inducing repigmentation of vitiligo lesions. The excimer lamp has a larger treatment field compared with excimer laser, which may enable irradiation of larger areas and shorter treatment times. Moreover, the cost of excimer lamp is cheaper compared with laser devices. Dose is given weekly and is based on MED.

Non-chromatic Ultraviolet Light Sources (Broadband 290–310 nm or Narrowband 313 nm)

These devices utilize fiberoptic systems coupled with UVB generating sources.

FACTORS AFFECTING TREATMENT PROTOCOLS

1. **Activity of vitiligo:** NB-UVB can be started regardless of disease activity, as it has both stabilizing and repigmenting effects; however, its repigmenting effects are less in active cases.
2. **Type of vitiligo:** Better responses are expected in cases with pigmented hairs and disease duration of 6 months or less.
3. **Skin phototype:** It is suggested that patients with darker skin phototype-III and higher are expected to achieve better response with phototherapy.
4. **Disease duration and hair color:** Poor responses might be encountered in long-standing lesions even when pigmented hairs are present. In such cases, combination with surgical procedures could be considered.
5. **Distribution of lesions:** The expected response rate varies from face, being most responsive to acral areas, being least responsive. Also amongst face, sites like pre- and post-auricular, lips, angles of mouth are less responsive. Similarly in hands, periungual areas are least responsive as compared to proximal areas. The reason for this anatomic variation in the response to treatment is still unclear, but may be attributed to the regional variation in the density of hair follicles, "the melanocytes reservoir."

6. **Patient's response to light:** History of photosensitivity or photo koebnerization should be ruled out before starting phototherapy.
7. **Special sites (genitals):** It has long been recommended to cover male genitals during the session; this was also the VWG consensus. However, the consensus did not mention how to manage lesions in the genital areas. Apart from an old report of malignancy developing at exposed genitals, no studies have further supported or ruled out the hazard of phototherapy to these sites. Thus, excimer light might be a useful suggested line, if topical treatment is not effective.

ADVERSE EFFECTS

Acute Effects

Acute side effects of phototherapy include sunburn-like reaction with erythema, which, depending on the severity, may be accompanied by tenderness, pruritus, and less commonly peeling and blistering of the skin. Tanning, xerosis, reactivation of herpes simplex, and injury to the eyes, if appropriate UV protective goggles are not worn during treatment and are also immediate side effects common to both UVB and UVA phototherapy.

PUVA has additional acute side effects which include nausea, headache, dizziness, and sunburn-like erythema reactions and acute ocular reaction secondary to additional sun exposure in the 24 hours following treatment, if photo protection and UVA-protective eyewear are not worn.

Long-Term Side Effects

Photoaging, actinic keratosis, and photo-carcinogenesis are long-term side effects of phototherapy and photochemotherapy.

With greater than 300 treatments, BB-UVB is associated with a modest but significant increase in squamous cell carcinoma (SCC) and basal cell carcinoma (BCC). However, the carcinogenic risk of a single PUVA treatment is about seven times greater than a single UVB treatment. The risk of non-melanoma skin cancer is dose-dependent with PUVA. Therefore, the maximum recommended lifetime exposure of PUVA is more than 250 treatments.

PROTECTION DURING PHOTOTHERAPY

While on phototherapy, there are a few things which should be kept in mind (Table 8.4).

COMMON OBSTACLES

Common obstacles faced during phototherapy are discussed below.

- *Arrest of repigmentation*: With phototherapy the exposed skin becomes thickened and lichenified, this is a type of photoadaptation. In such cases, a plateau is reached with arrest in further repigmentation. To overcome this, patient is advised to apply topical steroids and keratolytics.
- *Failure of repigmentation*: In some situations, lesions with a typically good prognosis fail to repigment. The solutions include checking the machine, patient's position in the chamber or additional therapy can be instituted.
- *New lesions developing while on treatment*: This should raise the suspicion of photo koebnerization, deeming this line of therapy an improper one.
- *Failure of compliance*: Successful treatment is directly related to patient compliance. If the patient cannot maintain a consistent schedule in phototherapy, other options should be considered.
- *Darkening of normal skin*: Perilesional skin becomes darker with phototherapy, making the lesions more obvious. To prevent this, unaffected skin should be covered or sunscreen can be applied.
- *Frequent development of marked erythema*: This can occur due to fixed high starting dose in some centres, uneven exposures (obesity) or ingestion of photosensitizer drugs before phototherapy.

COMPARISON OF EFFICACY AND RESULTS OF VARIOUS PHOTOTHERAPEUTIC MODALITIES

i. *NB-UVB versus PUVA*: In 1997, Westerhof and Nieuweboer-Krobotova were the first group that reported the efficacy of NB-UVB for vitiligo. They performed an observer-blinded prospective study comparing NB-UVB with topical PUVA. At 4 months, 46% (n = 13) of the patients treated with topical PUVA showed repigmentation compared to 67% (n = 52) of the patients treated with NB-UVB.

Table 8.4: Protection during phototherapy
While in the unit: • Eyes protected with small UV opaque goggles • Face protected using sunscreen or pillow-case • Male genitalia protected using jock-straps or underpants
After exposure to psoralens: Avoidance of sun-exposure • Eyes protected with goggles and skin with clothes, sunscreens until sunset
Non-treatment days: Avoid sun exposure and protect skin with sunscreens

Table 8.5: Combination therapies with NB-UVB

Drug	Efficacy on combination with NB-UVB		Study	Combination, %	NB-UVB, %	Combination advised or not
Topical steroids	Stabilization Significant increase in mean repig-mentation	Clobetasol	Lim-Ong et al, 2005	55	40	+
Topical calcineurin inhibitors	Results inferior to steroids Faster repigmentation when combi-ned with NB-UVB	Tacrolimus	Nordal et al, 2011	42	29	+
			Mehrabi and Pandya, 2006	49	41	–
			Satyanarayan et al, 2013	33	28	–
	Treatment efficacy is dose dependent	Pimecrolimus	Esfandiarpour et al, 2009	69	25	+
Topical vitamin D analogs	Contradictory results, no significant value vs rapid initiation of pigmentation on combina-tion with NB-UVB	Calcipotriol	Arca et al, 2006	46	42	+
		Tacalcitol	Leone et al, 2006	50	40	–
Antioxidants	Systemic antioxidants showed significant increase in mean pig-mentation area	Vitamin E	Elgoweini and Nour El Din, 2009	73	56	+
			Dell Anna et al, 2007	47	18	+
			Doghim et al, 2011	40	45	–
	Topical antioxidants showed no significant value in RCTs	CSOD gel	Yuskel et al, 2009	5	0	+/–

Abbreviations: CSOD—catalase superoxide dismutase, RCT: Randomized controlled trials

Since then many prospective clinical trials have been done and have demonstrated that NB-UVB has superior efficacy. Apart from its efficacy, NB-UVB has a better safety profile compared with PUVA, mainly due to absence of adverse effects related to psoralen.

ii. *NB-UVB versus 308 nm excimer laser and monochromatic excimer light*: Hong and colleagues found that excimer laser had greater efficacy compared with NB-UVB in the treatment of vitiligo, and induced more rapid and greater degree of repigmentation. Cassaci et al compared 308 nm monochromatic excimer light to NB-UVB in randomized, investigator blinded and half-side comparison trial and showed similar repigmentation rate in both. In addition, several recent meta-analyses also have shown similar efficacy between excimer light, excimer laser, and NB-UVB for the treatment of vitiligo.

iii. *BB-UVB versus NB-UVB and PUVA*: Since broadband-UVB has been largely replaced by NB-UVB, very limited evidence exists on the treatment of vitiligo with BB-UVB. A meta-analysis by Njoo et al compared data on BB-UVB, NB-UVB, and PUVA. Treatment was considered successful when more than 75% repigmentation was achieved. The highest success rates were achieved with NB-UVB (63%, with a 95% confidence interval ranging from 50–76%), followed by BB-UVB (57%, with a confidence interval ranging from 29–82%), and PUVA (51%, with a 95% confidence interval ranging from 46–56%).

COMBINATION THERAPY

Even though NB-UVB is the cornerstone treatment of vitiligo, combinations with medical and/or surgical therapies improve patients' odds in their battle against this disease. Over the years, several combination plans were suggested, some with proven efficacy, others with controversial results, and the rest were of denied value (Table 8.5). Combination therapies serve multiple purposes:

1. **Induction of stabilization:**
   - *Immunomodulation*: Systemic and topical steroids, immunosuppressants, topical calcineurin inhibitors and topical calcipotriol.
   - *Overcoming oxidative stress*: Oral and topical antioxidants.

2. **Enhancement of repigmentation:**
   - *Stimulation of melanogenesis*: Calcineurin inhibitors and vitamin D analogs.
   - *Improving the melanocyte environment for better migration*: Dermabrasion, fractional lasers.

3. **Supplying the missing reservoir:** Surgical techniques.

NEW HORIZONS IN THE TREATMENT OF VITILIGO

Developments in the phototherapy field are never ending, with newer machines, protocols, combinations, and evaluation techniques emerging to improve results and safety profiles, and expand the sector of patients with vitiligo who benefit from this line of treatment. Low-level laser therapy (LLLT) and home-based phototherapy are two such novel techniques.

Bibliography

1. Al Ghamdi KM, Kumar A, Moussa NA. Low-level laser therapy: a useful technique for enhancing the proliferation of various cultured cells. Lasers Med Sci 2012;27(1):237–49.

2. Arca E, Tastan HB, Erbil AH, et al. Narrow-band ultraviolet B as monotherapy and in combination with topical calcipotriol in the treatment of vitiligo. J Dermatol 2006;33:338–43.

3. Dell'Anna ML, Mastrofrancesco A, Sala R, et al. Antioxidants and narrow band-UVB in the treatment of vitiligo: a double-blind placebo controlled trial. Clin Exp Dermatol 2007;32: 631–6.

4. Doghim NN, Hassan AM, El-Ashmawy AA, et al. Topical antioxidant and narrowband versus topical combination of calcipotriol plus betamethathone dipropionate and narrowband in the treatment of vitiligo. Life Sci J 2011;8:186–97.

5. Elgoweini M, Nour El Din N. Response of vitiligo to narrowband ultraviolet B and oral antioxidants. J Clin Pharmacol 2009;49:852–5.

6. Esfandiarpour I, Ekhlasi A, Farajzadeh S, et al. The efficacy of pimecrolimus 1% cream plus narrowband ultraviolet B in the treatment of vitiligo: a double-blind, placebo-controlled clinical trial. J Dermatolog Treat 2009;20:14–8.

7. Grimes PE. Psoralen photochemotherapy for vitiligo. Clin Dermatol 1997;15(6):921–6.

8. Leone G, Pacifico A, Iacovelli P, et al. Tacalcitol and narrow-band phototherapy in patients with vitiligo. Clin Exp Dermatol 2006;31:200–5.

9. Lim-Ong M, Leveriza RM,OngBE, et al. Comparison between narrow-band UVB with topical corticosteroid and narrow-band UVB with placebo in the treatment of vitiligo: a randomized controlled trial. J Philipp Dermatol Soc 2005; 14:17–22.

10. Mehrabi D, Pandya AG. A randomized, placebocontrolled, doubleblind trial comparing narrowband UV-B plus 0.1% tacrolimus ointment with narrowband UV-B plus placebo in the treatment of generalized vitiligo. Arch Dermatol 2006;142: 927–9.

11. Millington GW , Levell NJ . Vitiligo: the historical curse of depigmentation. Int J Dermatol 2007; 46:990–995 .

12. Nordal EJ, Guleng GE, Ro¨nnevig JR. Treatment of vitiligo with narrowband- UVB (TL01) combined with tacrolimus ointment (0.1%) vs. placebo ointment, a randomized right/left double-blind comparative study. J Eur Acad Dermatol Venereol 2011;25:1440–3.

13. Roelandts R. The history of phototherapy: something new under the sun? J Am Acad Dermatol 2002;46:926–930.

14. Satyanarayan HS, Kanwar AJ, Parsad D, et al. Efficacy and tolerability of combined treatment with NB-UVB and topical tacrolimus versus NBUVB alone in patients with vitiligo vulgaris: a randomized intra-individual open comparative trial. Indian J Dermatol Venereol Leprol 2013;79: 525–7.

15. Shan X, Wang C, Tian H, et al. Narrow-band ultraviolet B home phototherapy in vitiligo. Indian J Dermatol Venereol Leprol 2014;80(4):336–8.

16. Westerhof W, Nieuweboer-Krobotova L. Treatment of vitiligo with UV-B radiation vs topical psoralen plus UV-A. Arch Dermatol 1997; 133(12): 1525–8.

17. Yuksel EP, Aydin F, Senturk N, et al. Comparison of the efficacy of narrow band ultraviolet B and narrow band ultraviolet B plus topical catalase-superoxide dismutase treatment in vitiligo patients. Eur J Dermatol 2009;19:341–4.

Rational Use of Triple Combination Creams

Arijit Coondoo

Topical corticosteroids (TCs) are a unique set of drugs which are beneficially prescribed for a large number of skin ailments. They were introduced in 1952 when Sulzberger and Witten first reported the utility of corticosteroids on topical application. The basic chemical structure of the TC introduced by them was a pregnane ring comprising a cyclic hydrocarbon with four ring structures of three hexane rings and one pentane ring. This structure was subsequently repeatedly modified to yield newer TCs with varied potencies and efficacy.

How to use Topical Corticosteroids?

Though TCs were initially introduced as anti-inflammatory medications, they were also reported to have anti-proliferative and immunosuppressive properties. TCs have, therefore, been prescribed in various eczematous disorders such as atopic dermatitis and contact dermatitis, papulosquamous disorders such as psoriasis and lichen planus, connective tissue disorders, bullous disorders, pigmentary disorders, neutrophilic disorders, mucous membrane disorders, cutaneous malignancies and other conditions where they can reduce inflammation. However, they are contraindicated in infections (fungal, bacterial, viral, etc.), on ulcerated skin or when the patient has hypersensitivity to TCs. According to their efficacy and potency, the corticosteroids are divided into 7 groups (USA classification), with the potency decreasing gradually from Class I to Class VII (*see* Appendix).

TCs should be used with extreme caution in the soft skin of infants and children, on the face, groin and axilla and also in the geriatric age group and in pregnancy. Hence, a thorough knowledge about the potency of a TC is of utmost importance not only to determine its dermatological indications, but also to assess its suitability of use in the special situations mentioned above. Indiscriminate use may lead to dermatological and systemic side effects, some of which may be irreversible. The wide variety of indications and easy availability of TCs have caused them to be the victims of a significant amount of abuse and misuse in recent times.

How Topical Corticosteroids are Misused?

Misuse of TCs in India is gradually increasing. The misuse occurs at various levels. Pharmaceutical companies manufacture irrational combinations of TCs with other molecules completely disregarding the norms for judicious use of the drug. One glaring example is the so-called "modified Kligman's regime". This triple combination of hydroquinone, tretinoin and TC is promoted by salespersons for use in melasma. The original combination which was discovered by Kligman et al. in 1974 contained a low potent TC. However, most of these newer combinations contain mometasone, a mid-potent TC which may cause harm to the face. Salespersons of pharmaceuticals also promote TCs by explaining their advantages in glowing terms while keeping the cautions and side effects under the wraps. Promotion of TCs is made not only to doctors but also practitioners of alternative medicines and quacks. While the latter are also frequent prescribers of TCs, patients also tend to buy TCs from chemists after the drug is "recommended" by friends, neighbors and relatives, salesmen at chemist's shops, beauticians and other laymen. A study conducted in 12 centers of dermatology spread across the country (Saraswat A et al.) found that 59.3% of patients were using TC on the face without any doctor's prescription. Of the remainder, only 26.7% patients had used TC prescribed by a dermatologist. Adding to the problem is the fact that all TCs are sold as OTC products resulting in easy availability at all sales counters of chemists. Patients may purchase TCs without any prescription or by repeating the same prescription over and over again. A recent phenomenon of equating certain TCs with fairness creams has increased sales of TCs but compounded the incidence of ill-effects of TC misuse. Thus injudicious use of TCs occurs through various avenues. Such abuse of TC does not take into account any of the precautionary measures regarding TC prescription and exposes the user to the disastrous effects of overuse and abuse of TCs.

Effects of TC Misuse

TC misuse leads to various physical and psychological disturbance. Physically, it can cause a large number of side effects which may be local or systemic.

Local Effects

The local side effects are atrophy and striae, acneiform eruptions, secondary infections such as tinea incognito, hypopigmentation (the basis for its use as a fairness cream), hypertrichosis, telangiectasia, erythema, purpura, bruises, ulcers and allergic contact dermatitis.

Systemic Effects

Systemic side effects include adrenal suppression (particularly after overuse of potent TCs), growth retardation in children, glaucoma and cataracts (if potent and mid-potent TCs are used around eyes) and hyperglycemia.

Psychological Effects

The psychological side effects are TC addiction and TC phobia. TC addiction (dependence) results from repeated and prolonged use of potent or mid-potent TCs. The patient experiences psychological distress on stoppage of the drug. Stopping the drug can also result in the rebound phenomenon affecting the face, genitalia and other parts of the body. As mentioned earlier, a multicentric study of this phenomenon on the face found severe manifestations of steroid dependence which were collectively named as topical steroid dependent faces (TSDF). TC phobia, on the other hand, implies a fear of using TCs. It has been observed in particular among parents of children suffering from atopic dermatitis, a condition where the use of TCs is therapeutically imperative.

How to Minimize TC Misuse?

Various steps have been suggested to stop TC misuse. Some of these are:

1. Stopping manufacture of unethical combinations of TC by pharmaceuticals.
2. Stopping advertisements of potent and superpotent TCs in lay press and electronic media by pharmaceuticals.
3. Enacting a law to enforce a ban on the non-prescription sale of TC.
4. Stopping sale of TCs by repeating prescriptions.
5. Restriction on the sale of TCs prescribed by practitioners of alternative medicines and quacks.
6. Taking bureaucratic and other regulatory steps for strict implementation of such a law.
7. Taking effective steps to sensitize the government regarding the evils of TC misuse.
8. Intensive campaign to increase awareness of TC misuse among the lay public as well as medical professionals. Such a campaign should be conducted in the print media, electronic media as well as at a personal level by dermatologists during their interaction with patients. However, such a campaign should be balanced judiciously so that it does not cause TC phobia in the minds of the target community members.

The Indian Association of Dermatologists, Venereologists and Leprologists (IADVL) has already started taking measures to implement the above suggestions. Following a proposal to this effect passed in 2007, a study was conducted in 2008 at 12 centers spread across India on the ill-effects of such a misuse on the face. The startling results of the study were published in 2011. While dermatologists have been individually campaigning against TC misuse, a symposium to this effect was published in 2014 in the Indian Journal of Dermatology. The IADVL has also set up a committee named the IADVL committee against topical steroid misuse (ITATSA) to campaign against TC misuse in 2014.

Bibliography

1. Coondoo A, Phiske M, Verma S, Lahiri K. Side-effects of topical steroids: A long overdue revisit. Indian Dermatology Online J 2014;5:416–25.

2. Coondoo A. Topical steroid misuse: The Indian scenario. Indian J Dermatol 2014;59:451–5.

3. Ghosh A, Sengupta S, Coondoo A, Jana A. Topical corticosteroid addiction and phobia. Indian J Dermatol 2014;59: 465–468.

4. Goa KL. Clinical pharmacology and pharmacokinetic properties of topically applied corticosteroids. A review. Drugs 1988; 36 Suppl 5: 51–61.

5. Kligman AM, Willis I. A new formula for depigmenting human skin. Arch Dermatol 1975;111:40–8.

6. Saraswat A, Lahiri K, Chatterjee M, Barua S, Coondoo A, et at. Topical corticosteroid abuse on the face: A prospective, multicenter study of dermatology outpatients. Indian J Dermatol Venereol Leprol 2011 Mar Apr; 77(2): 160–6.

7. Sulzberger MB, Witten VH. The effect of topically applied compound F in selected dermatoses. J Invest Dermatol 1952; 19(2): 101–2.

Acne Vulgaris in Pigmented Skin

Kabir Sardana

Acne vulgaris (AV) in skin of color shares many of the clinical features typically seen in lighter skin types. However, concomitant postinflammatory hyperpigmentation (PIH) is a key distinguishing feature of acne in the darker-skinned patient (Figs 10.1 and 10.2). This is a cause of cosmetic concern. Patients frequently refer to the lesions of PIH as scars, and the cosmetic disfigurement caused by PIH adds to the psychological distress associated with acne.

Another reason is that patients tend to manipulate the lesions and the excoriated lesions typically appear as hypopigmented macules with hyperpigmented borders (Fig. 10.3). This is seen commonly in females (Fig. 10.4).

In India, a common cause is the use of corticosteroid-containing skin bleaching products (e.g. Lobate, Betnovate, Skin Lite, etc.). Another cause is the use of cosmetics and facial foundations. Ideally occlusive skin products should be avoided. Also comedogenic makeups (e.g. when used to mask hyperpigmentation) can actually cause more acne and more PIH.

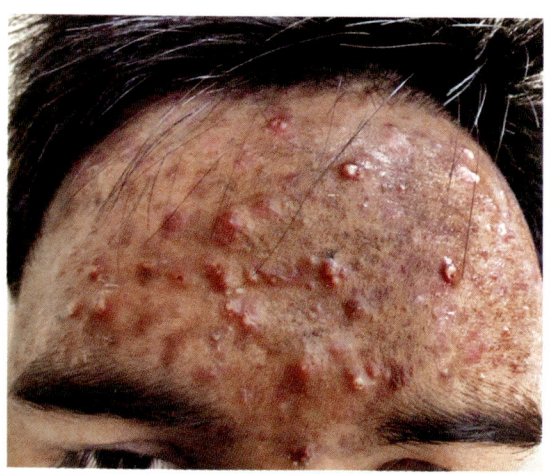

Fig. 10.1: An admixture of papules, pustules, nodules and pigmentation (moderate grade acne)

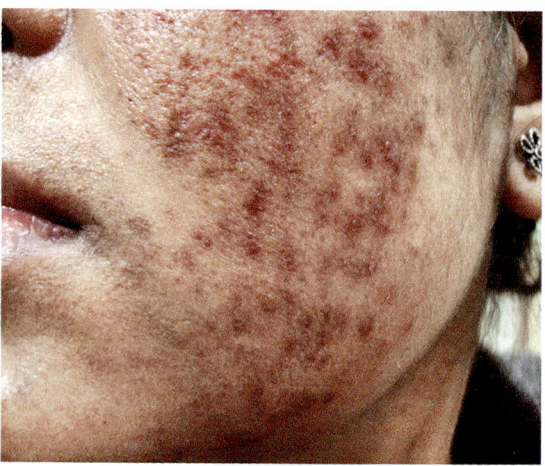

Fig. 10.2: A female patient with persistent pigmentation following healing of acne lesions

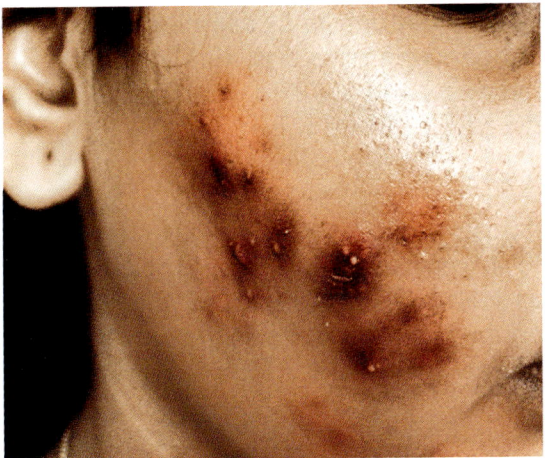

Fig. 10.3: A female patient with acne with sequelae of compulsive "picking"

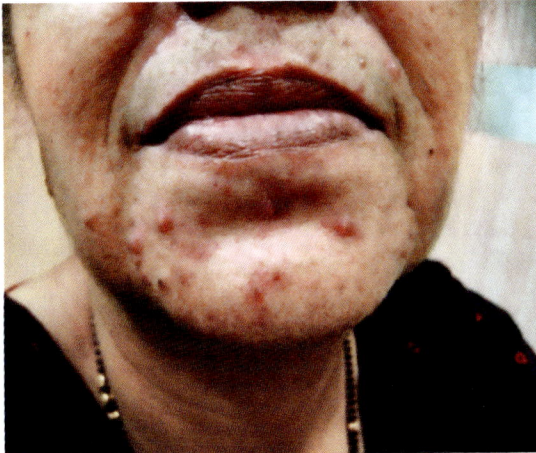

Fig. 10.4: Perioral dermatitis in a female patients

TREATMENT PRINCIPLES

The basic principles are listed in Table 10.1.

Topical Agents

Retinoids

They target hyperkeratinization and comedogenesis and possess anti-inflammatory and antifibrotic properties. Most importantly they are capable of reducing hyperpigmentation by inhibiting tyrosinase, inhibiting melanosome transfer, dispersing epidermal melanin, and promoting desquamation which leads to removal of epidermal melanin.

a. Tolerability depends on concentration, dosing, and vehicle, all of which must be taken into account when selecting a retinoid. When using tazarotene or generic tretinoin, always use A CREAM vehicle as they are less likely to cause drying and irritation. Some microsphere can also be used.

Table 10.1: Overview of therapy in acne
Reduce inflammation
• Initiate effective and appropriately aggressive treatment early in disease course
• Include topical BPO and topical retinoid in treatment regimen
• Low threshold to initiate oral antibiotics when indicated
Minimize irritation
• Treatment regimen must be well tolerated
• Appropriate selection of vehicle, concentration and dosing
• Gradual change of vehicle, concentration, and dosing as tolerated
Eliminate exacerbating factors
• Use silicone-based hair products and noncomedogenic cosmetics (e.g. mineral makeups) and moisturizers
• Apply hair products at least 1 inch, behind hairline or limit application to distal hair shafts
Educate patient about PIH
• Difference between active acne lesions and PIH
• Establish realistic expectation regarding treatment outcome (e.g. length of treatment), potential need for adjunctive treatments for PIH
• Importance of sun protection

b. Short contact application or alternate-night application is appropriate in patients who cannot tolerate nightly application; application time is gradually increased as tolerated. The concentration can also be increased as tolerated, usually after at least 4–6 weeks of treatment with the lower strength.

c. For retinoid-naive patients, a good practice is to initiate with: Adapalene 0.1% gel or cream, tretinoin 0.025% or 0.05% cream or 0.04% gel (when a branded microsphere formulation is used), or tazarotene 0.05% cream.

d. In addition, patients should be advised to use gentle cleansers and moisturizers with sunscreen and discontinue all harsh and potentially irritating skin products, especially astringents and exfoliating treatments that may increase their sensitivity to topical retinoids.

BPO

Benzoyl peroxide (BPO) and topical antibiotics are also important in the management of AV. Similar to retinoids, the primary consideration when selecting an antimicrobial agent is maximizing efficacy while minimizing irritation and the potential for pigment alteration.

Though there is a unique advantage of BPO in preventing resistance, there is an issue of irritation that can lead to pigmentation. An ideal combination is BPO 5% clindamycin 1% gel plus tretinoin 0.04% gel. As stated above, while benzoyl peroxide is safe and effective in patients with skin of color, caution is advised to minimize irritation—which could result in postinflammatory pigment alteration.

Thus a simple method to avoid PIH is to use benzoyl peroxide in concentrations of 5% or less for the face. In fact 2.5% is ideal. Another option is to use a fixed combination product. Adapalene 0.1% and benzoyl peroxide 2.5% in an aqueous gel has also been studied in subjects with skin of color.

Another option is to use nadifloxacin or clindamycin (this has high resistance in India) gel and use it in combination with a benzoyl peroxide wash.

Azelaic Acid

Azelaic acid 20% cream has also been found to successfully treat acne and is as effective as tretinoin 0.05% cream, BPO 5% gel, erythromycin 2% ointment, and clindamycin 1% gel. Like BPO, *P. acnes* resistance to azelaic acid has not been reported. Azelaic acid is well tolerated and relatively mild, so it is a suitable option for individuals with sensitive skin. It appears to have an inhibitory effect on melanocyte proliferation and melanogenesis, so it can potentially reduce hyperpigmentation. It is a especially useful treatment option for skin of color patients with PIH who cannot tolerate retinoids. Greater efficacy and patient satisfaction have been reported with various topical combination regimens containing azelaic acid compared to monotherapy.

- In my view, the problem is that the quality of azelaic acid base in India is not good enough thus most AZA products are not as good as topical antibiotics, topical benzoyl peroxide formulations or retinoids.

- Topical dapsone 5% gel is a sulfone in aqueous gel that has been recently approved in India. Clinical trial data and clinical experience suggest that dapsone 5% gel is well tolerated and no racial/ethnic differences in safety have been identified. Therefore, topical dapsone should also be considered an appropriate therapeutic option in the topical management of AV in skin of color patients. Again in India, the base of the available dapsone gel is not good enough

Oral Therapy

For patients with moderate-to-severe acne, systemic therapy may be required to achieve

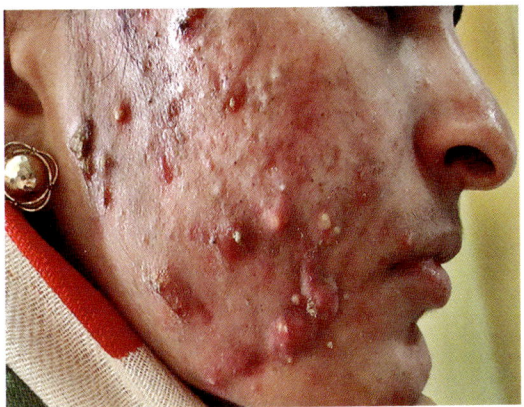

Fig. 10.5: A female patient with nodules and cysts. Such case should warrant investigation for an underlying disorder

satisfactory results. Oral treatments consist of antibiotics, retinoids, and hormonal modulators. In skin of color patients, a lower threshold to initiate oral treatment is recommended in order to reduce inflammation at an earlier stage, thus reducing the risk of PIH and scarring.

In females with hormonal acne, it will be advisable to treat with hormonal agents (Fig. 10.5).

Author prefers a low dose isotretinoin even as low as 5 mg alternate day can help to avoid irritation and prevent PIH.

Procedural Therapies

In-office procedures are often utilized as adjunctive therapeutic options for AV. Two well-established and widely used procedures are comedone extraction and intralesional corticosteroids. Their key advantages are that they do not require any anesthesia, do not have any associated "downtime" or significant post-procedure care, and quickly lead to resolution of targeted lesions. An overview of various therapy options for various scars and sequelae are listed in Figs 10.6 to 10.9.

- Comedone extraction, or acne surgery, reduces comedones, both open and closed, by pushing out the follicular plug. Topical retinoids may make the lesions more amenable to extraction, and a 6–8 weeks course prior to the procedure is recommended in skin of color patients to help reduce trauma and PIH.
- Intralesional corticosteroids (e.g. triamcinolone acetonide 2.5–5.0 mg/cc) can be used to treat inflammatory lesions. Improvement is usually noted within 2–5 days. These "quick fix" treatments are often beneficial in patients with skin of color to prevent progression to larger lesions or the development of negative sequelae.
- Superficial chemical peels can be used to treat both acne and PIH, but deep chemical peels are not recommended in patients with skin of color as they are associated with a greater risk of scarring

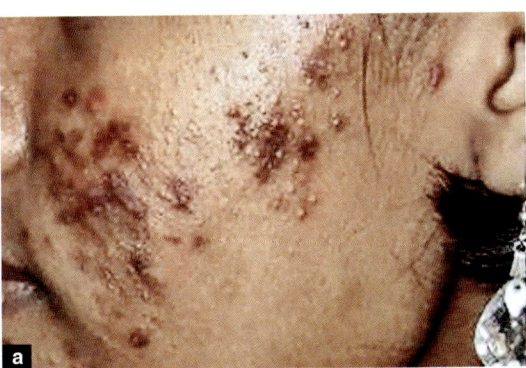
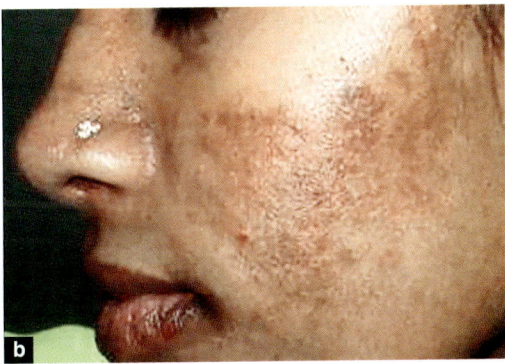

Fig. 10.6: Macular hyperpigmented scars treated with salicylic acid chemical peels: (a) Before treatment; (b) After treatment

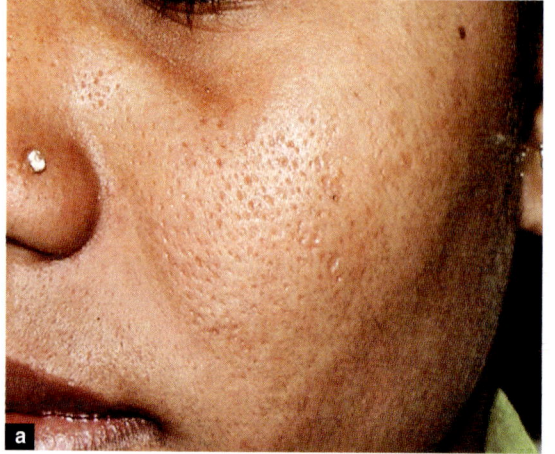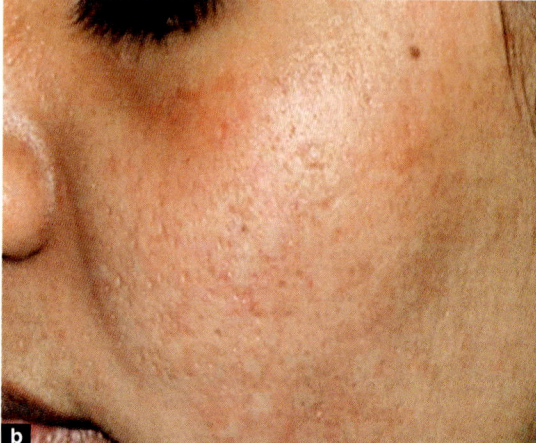

Fig. 10.7: Icepick scars: (a) Before treatment; (b) After treatment

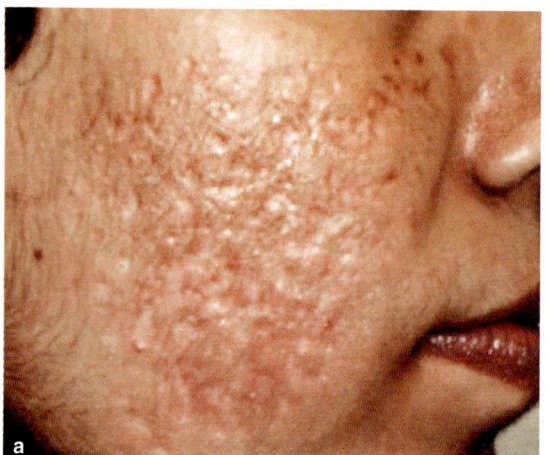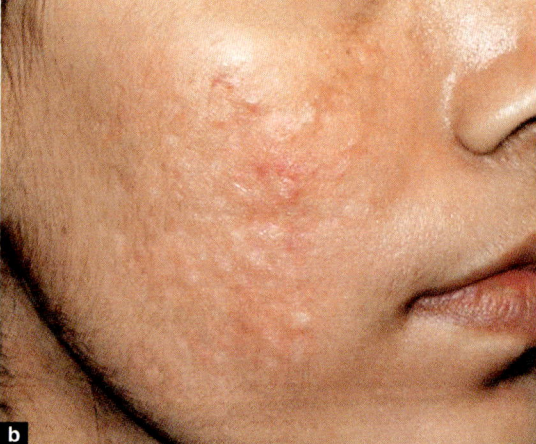

Fig. 10.8: Rolling scars treated with subcision and microneedling: (a) Before treatment; (b) After treatment

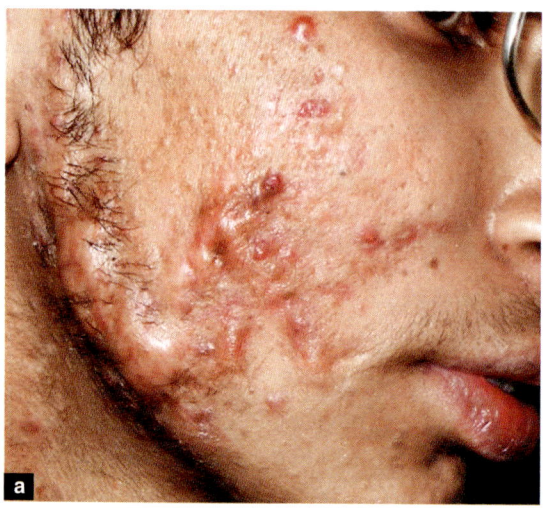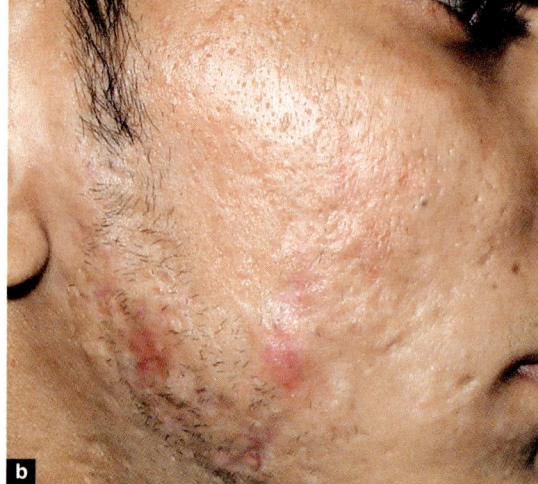

Fig. 10.9: Hypertrophic scars treated with intralesional steroids: (a) Before treatment; (b) After treatment

and PIH. Superficial chemical peels include salicylic acid 20–30%, glycolic acid 20–70%, trichloroacetic acid 10–35%, and Jessner's peel. In the author's experience, salicylic acid peels are the preferred choice for patients with both acne and PIH. Grimes investigated the safety and efficacy of 20–30% salicylic acid peels performed every 2 weeks in 25 patients (skin types V and VI) with various conditions including acne and PIH.

• Light, laser, and photodynamic treatments have been studied but conservative settings should be used to avoid side effects. They may not be very useful as a monotherapy for PIH.

Bibliography

1. Alexis AF, Sergay AB, Taylor SC. Common dermatologic disorders in skin of color: a comparative practice survey. Cutis 2007;80(5):387–94.

2. Child FJ, Fuller LC, Higgins EM, Du Vivier AW. A study of the spectrum of skin disease occurring in a black population in south-east London. Br J Dermatol 1999;141(3):512–7.

3. Halder RM, Grimes PE, McLaurin CI, Kress MA, Kenney Jr JA. Incidence of common dermatoses in a predominantly black dermatologic practice. Cutis 1983;32(4):388–90.

4. Halder RM, Holmes YC, Bridgeman-Shah S, Kligman A. A clinical pathological study of acnevulgaris in black females. J Invest Dermatol 1996;106:888.

5. Hongcharu W, Taylor CR, Chang Y, Aghassi D, Suthamjariya K, Anderson RR. Topical ALA-photodynamic therapy for the treatment of acne vulgaris. J Invest Dermatol 2000;115(2): 183–92.

6. Sardana K, Chugh S, Garg VK. The role of zinc in acne and prevention of resistance: have we missed the "base" effect? Int J Dermatol 2014 Jan; 53(1): 125–7. doi: 10.1111/ijd.12264. PubMed PMID: 24350859.

7. Sardana K, Garg VK. Low-dose isotretinoin in acne vulgaris: a critical review. Br J Dermatol 2011 Sep;165(3):698-700. doi: 10.1111/j.1365–2133.2011.10440.x. Epub 2011 Aug 4. PubMed PMID: 21623757.

8. Sardana K, Gupta T, Garg VK, Ghunawat S. Antibiotic resistance to Propionobacterium acnes: worldwide scenario, diagnosis and management. Expert Rev Anti Infect Ther 2015 Jul;13(7):883-96. doi: 10.1586/14787210.2015.1040765. Epub 2015 May 29. Review. PubMed PMID: 26025191.

9. Sardana K, Gupta T, Kumar B, Gautam HK, Garg VK. Cross-sectional Pilot Study of Antibiotic Resistance in Propionibacterium Acnes Strains in Indian Acne Patients Using 16S-RNA Polymerase Chain Reaction: A Comparison Among Treatment Modalities Including Antibiotics, Benzoyl Peroxide, and Isotretinoin. Indian J Dermatol 2016 Jan-Feb;61(1):45–52. doi: 10.4103/0019-5154.174025. PubMed PMID: 26955094; PubMed Central PMCID: PMC4763694.

10. Sardana K, Gupta T, Kumar B, Gautam HK. Efficacy of a single daily dose of levofloxacin in gram-negative folliculitis complicating acne vulgaris. Skin Med 2015 Dec 1;13(6):488-90. eCollection 2015. PubMed PMID: 26861531.

11. Sardana K, Singh C, Narang I, Bansal S, Garg VK. The role of antimullerian hormone in the hormonal workup of women with persistent acne. J Cosmet Dermatol 2016 Dec;15(4):343-349. doi: 10.1111/jocd.12235. Epub 2016 Jun 20. PubMed PMID: 27320497.

12. Sardana K, Verma G. Propionibacterium acnes and the Th1/Th17 Axis, Implications in Acne Pathogenesis and Treatment. Indian J Dermatol 2017 Jul-Aug;62(4):392–394. doi: 10.4103/ijd.IJD_483_16. PubMed PMID: 28794550; PubMed Central PMCID: PMC5527720.

Dark Is Beautiful

Nandita Das

How it all Began?

The *'Dark is beautiful'* campaign was launched by an organization called Women of Worth, headed by Kavitha Emmanuel. Many think that I started the campaign, but I am just happy that it has created a debate around the issue which should have happened many years ago. I got to know about them when she contacted me to lend support to the campaign. Of course I was glad to, as it is a discrimination that is rampant, across class and region and now, even gender! The imageries all around are perpetuating and promoting this stereotype. So while it was all around me, I had not given it focused attention, till I started supporting the campaign. I did not realize the magnitude of the damage the prejudice and the combined impact of products and imageries were having on young minds.

The "Fair is Fabulous" mindset and the message "Dark is Beautiful" gives out: The "Fair is Beautiful" mindset has reached bizarre levels with vagina washes to make the woman's private parts fair for the husband! How much worse can it get? Every skin care product is promoted with the fairness element in it. The real dangerous messaging is that only fairness will make you successful/beautiful/acceptable/loved.

Too many young girls and now boys are losing their confidence purely because of a prejudice that discriminates. They are being made to feel unworthy, inadequate, unacceptable. I think the campaign, "Dark Is Beautiful", is trying to say that be comfortable in your skin, even if the world around you tells you that you are not good enough, if you are not fair.

We are defined by what we do, how we think and respond to situations and not by born identities like cast, religion, nationality or the color of our skin. We have no hand in them, so why feel proud or ashamed about it. The campaign is trying to draw attention to the obsession with fairness and how it is destroying the self-esteem of millions of people, especially young girls.

Importance of Campaign and the Extent of It

There are many campaigns that I support. Very recently I have supported campaigns for organ donations, signed petitions against genetically modified crops and to save the RTI from being wrongly amended. And this one that tells you to be comfortable in your skin is only one of them. I have always been very outspoken about this issue, but till recently it was more informal. The issue of dark skin would always pop-up in the many things I did, but did not take center stage. I am so glad that such a campaign has been launched and I am able to add my voice to it. As the issue impacts so many people, young girls in particular, by default I have become a champion of it!

I believe it is important to speak up and add one's voice to campaigns that are for the larger good. After all we are nothing but a drop in the ocean, but we do need every drop to fill it! So I will continue advocating what I believe in, both formally and informally, but there is no design or plan for it.

Impact

When I had supported this campaign, like I have done for many other campaigns, I did not realize that it would go viral. I was also clueless about it as I am not on the social media. I have been getting a lot of emails on the id that is on my website where mostly women, have shared their stories of discrimination and feel validated with this campaign.

The response has truly been overwhelming. I think the time had come to react to this fairness obsession.

I have talked about this at many forums, formally and informally. And I will continue to do so. This media interest will not last forever and nor will the campaign, but it would have triggered a debate that will have many tangible and intangible repercussions. I already see the ripples! To change a mindset takes time, but even baby steps in the right direction are needed.

Discrimination in Bollywood

I have had directors/camerapersons telling me that it would be good if I made my skin lighter as I was playing an educated upper class woman! If I get told all this, despite most people knowing my stand, I wonder what the other dark women are subjected to! Without exception, I have stood my ground, as I really do feel comfortable in my skin...literally! I would be told by the make-up man that I need not worry as he was an expert in making people look fair.

The glorification of the fair skin has been there in our films for a very long time. This reflects the bias of the society. In subtle and blatant ways, our language has things like, 'uska rang saafhai' for fair people as if the dark skin is dirty! It is tough to combat a mindset that finds many manifestations in our Indian songs, stories, myths and fables.

In Bollywood, most times, if you are dark, then you are right for the role of a village women, slum dweller, etc. but an urban affluent character always must be the fair faced person! Today the independent films thankfully deal with stories that are more real and edgy, and often about those who are marginalized. And as the characters are more realistic, there is really no need to put on too much make up and we can actually be ourselves.

Mainstream cinema, by its very definition, wants to appeal to the maximum number of people and if the society itself is deeply biased towards the fair skin then obviously all its reflections will have the same bias. While the bias exists in the society, the films, TV soaps, ads, etc. can play an important role in not further stereotyping what is 'beautiful'. Instead of breaking down these harmful notions that are destroying many a young women...and men, they are further associating fairness with success, love, marriage and over all acceptability by the world. While things have gotten worse with many more fairness products and the demand for the fairer skin may have gone up, but then it was not too different before.

The aesthetic sensibility is only a manifestation of the lack of respect for women as individuals. As long as women are objectified, they will be forced to buy into this story, that only if they were more "white/thin/beautiful" they would have a better chance in life, or that they would be good enough for this world. I believe such campaigns, debates, education and true empowerment of women will change things slowly.

There are many songs that equate fairness with beauty and pretty much all the heroines have been fair skinned. Same goes for the actors, who have done both independent and mainstream films, have had to lighten their skin for the latter. One knows this by the way the same actors look quite different in the two kinds of films!

Each one has a responsibility, individually and collectively as a Group because what we put out as a film industry impacts millions. It is for each person to decide what they should or should not do. No one can pass judgment, but one hopes that each of us will have a social conscience that will guide us to act more responsibly. Those in the public domain have a large circle of influence and we cannot undermine the impact it has on people. Sadly images that lower people's self esteem is deeply harmful to their well-being and I am sure no one would want that.

Men and the Fairness Obsession

I do get often asked about my reaction to men joining the race. But how is it any different? Why have we ignored it for so long? Till recently it was mostly women who were subjected to this 'you are not good enough if you are dark', but as looks for almost all have become more important than many other aspirations, men have joined the fray too. I find it strange when people say, "I am not an activist. My job is to entertain/ to make money/or to sing/dance or act". To be ethical and responsible beings, one does not have to be an activist. To not harm anyone's self esteem or to be mindful about one's impact is a way of thinking and living. I cannot believe that any sensible and sensitive person does not understand the repercussion such imageries and advertisements would have on young and vulnerable minds, but I guess the monies are big and people lose perspective. That is why it is important to have dialogue and debates around issues like this, in the public space. I do not want to sound judgmental, but I do not think it is such a difficult thing to do.

Root Cause of the 'Dark Skin Complex'

There are many theories for the fair skin obsession. But the one that seems most plausible is that of the caste hierarchy, which overlaps with the class pyramid. For centuries, the upper class/caste has been fair and the lower caste/working class, dark. The former works indoors and has had the best nutrition while the latter toils in the sun and is under privileged in many ways. With mixed marriages over centuries, we have a diverse variety in the way people look. But instead of celebrating the diversity, we as a nation have become obsessed about only being fair, as that represents power, wealth and privileges.

The films and ad companies are only cashing on the dark skin complex that already exists all across the country. While none of us have the right to dictate how others should behave, one cannot help wishing that the imageries that we see around ourselves would be truly representative of the diversity we see in the real world. The media are creating a furore about the attractiveness of white/fair skin, luring the dark-skinned individual into buying a product that will put them in the 'attractive' slot.

So it would not be wrong to say that the industry and media are working hand-in-glove in victimizing the customer who is nothing more than a consumer to them. However, when it is one's own individual choice then it is different, as I am all for freedom of choice. But this is about a mindset of society that puts pressure on the individual to be in a certain way, so that she/he is acceptable. This is about making someone feel inadequate, robbing them of their self-esteem. I think each one of us needs to be comfortable in our skin, even if the world around us tells us we are not good enough.

I do wish that people in influential positions would use their power for the larger good, to make people feel better about themselves and not to make them feel inadequate. Finally each one of us are guided by our own conscience and our inner sense of responsibility. The responsibility is primarily on each individual and thereby the society at large, but those who control its representations can be more responsible, so that they do not perpetuate this complex and instead help in breaking the stereotype. But, as the ad world is guided by money, they are only cashing on the aspirations of the consumer.

Has My Skin Color been the Reason for not Getting Commercial Offers?

The dark color is surely a handicap for mainstream films, but as my own interest has not been in commercial films, I have not had to fight that battle. Commercial industry is not for me, for many reasons and one of them is the stereotyping of most things. If you see, all the actors who were somewhat darker in their first film, are now, all fair.

The pressure must be enormous to fit it. I have always stood up against this stereotype. And if they wanted a fairer woman for the part, I always say that they did the wrong casting!

"Dark and Dusky" does this Description Annoy Me?

When I am written about, I am often described as 'dark and dusky'. I do not object at all. I am all for calling a spade a spade. In fact dark does not need to be even softened to dusky! All I wonder is why is there a need to describe me through the color of my skin, as I believe there is more to me! Or is it simply because it is rather rare for a female actor to be dark and, therefore, it becomes imperative to make a point about it.

Any person's complexion is only one of its many features or characteristics and, therefore, to give it undue importance would be to do injustice to the person. That's all. While writing about me as an actor or my involvement in social issues, I see no pressing need to comment on the skin color. This is in reference to a context, where there has been an overt preference for the fair skin for centuries, and therefore, it is important that we go deeper into its impact on people's well-being. I am lucky that my parents did not instil any kind of complex, but I have seen hundreds of young girls losing their confidence and developing low self-esteem because of being dark.

Is the International Film Industry Different?

Well, I have done a few projects with international producers, and there has been no pressure to change my skin color. In fact, their make-up artists love our kind of tan and tend to do minimal makeup. Actually, when I go to the West, especially Europe, they love our skin color. The obsession with fairness is in most Asian and African countries. With globalization, we also transfer complexes and the market forces make the most of it by creating an aspiration, here for instance, to be fair. Now even global brands are shamelessly advertising and selling fairness creams. It is human to like what one does not have, but those who are comfortable with who they are, do not feel the need to be someone else. The perception here is that if you need a lower class or lower caste character, then being dark is just what they want!

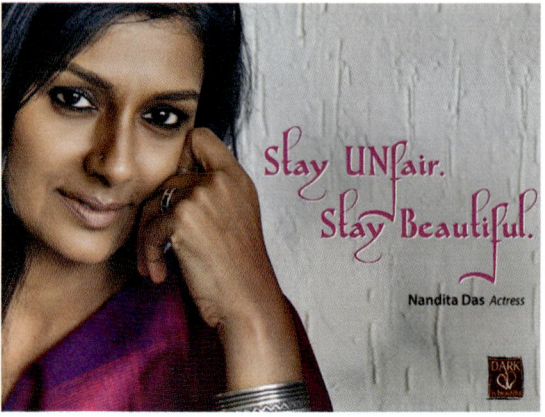

Nandita Das *Actress*

Personal Experience

As far as 'Dark is Beautiful', is concerned, I am directly connected to the cause. As a child, some distant relative would tell me not to go out in the sun lest I became darker, or when I walked into a store that had cosmetics, salespersons would come to me with the best anti-tan or fairness cream, or I would be told by the make-up man that I need not worry as he was an expert in making people look fair. I have even had directors/camerapersons telling me that it

would be good, if I made my skin lighter as I was playing an educated upper class woman!

Advice for Younger People and Women

Be yourself and be comfortable in your skin. Don't let anybody rob you off your self-esteem. Focus on your interests and talents and do things that make you happy, instead of making your looks the focal point of your identity. Let your attitude and behaviour define you and not just whatever you are born with. Stay natural, stay beautiful.

Appendix

We will cover steroids as they are possibly the most common drugs misused. The first part lists the topical steroids in the order of their potency from high potent (Class 1) to least potent (Class 7). Some commonly used brand names are given, though they do not reflect any commercial affiliations.

TOPICAL STEROIDS

A list of commonly used steroids is given below (Table A1). The milder steroids Class 6/7 are to be used for mild dermatoses, children, face/groin and for long-term usage. The potent steroids (Class 1, 2) are to be used either for severe dermatoses, adults, scalp, palm and soles for short durations. The mid-potent steroids can be used for longer periods, but with chronic use >6 weeks, all can cause side effects.

Highly responsive diseases will usually respond to weak steroid preparations, whereas less-responsive diseases require medium or high-potency topical steroids. Low-potent preparations should be used on the face and intertriginous areas. Very potent corticosteroids frequently under occlusion are usually required on hyper-

Table A1:	Equivalent doses of commonly used steroids	
Potency class	Chemical composition (concentration)	Common brand names
Class 7: Least potent	Hydrocortisone 0.5, 0.1, 2.5% preparations	Cutisoft (hydrocortisone 1%)
Class 6: Low potent	Fluocinolone acetonide 0.01% C, S desonide 0.05% C	Flucort lotion, Ultiderm lotion Desowen cream
Class 5: Lower mid-strength	Fluocinolone acetonide 0.025% C Betamethasone dipropionate 0.05% L Fluticasone propionate 0.05% C Hydrocortisone 17 butyrate 0.1% C, O, S Betamethasone valerate 0.1% C	Flucort cream, Flucort Forte lotion Diprovate plus lotion Flutivate cream Shcorty H 17 Betnovate cream (Betnovate C, N, GM), Fucibet
Class 4: Mid-strength	Fluocinolone acetonide 0.01%, 0.025% O Halcinonide 0.025% C Clobetasone butyrate 0.05% C Desoximetasone 0.05% C Mometasone furoate 0.1% C, L Hydrocortisone aceponate 0.127% C	NA NA Eumosone Xinasone Momate Efficort*

(Contd.)

Table A1: Equivalent doses of commonly used steroids (*Contd.*)		
Potency class	*Chemical composition (concentration)*	*Common brand names*
Class 3: Upper mid-strength	Fluocinonide 0.05% Betamethasone dipropionate 0.05% C Betamethasone valerate 0.1% O Fluticasone propionate 0.005% O Halometasone 0.05% cream	N N Betnovate (S) Flutivate ointment, Flutibact Execare*
Class 2: High potent	Fluocinonide 0.05% C, O, G, S Desoximetasone 0.25% C, 0.5% G Betamethasone dipropionate 0.05% O Mometasone furoate 0.1% O	NA Dexomet, Xinasone HP Diprovate Momate
Class 1: Superpotent	Fluocinoide 0.1% C Clobetasol propionate 0.05% C, O, G, S, F Halobetasol propionate 0.05% C, O	Flucort H Tenovate, Topinate Halox

C cream, O ointment, G gel, S solution, F foam, L Lotion
*British National Formulary

Table A2: Responsiveness of dermatoses to topical application of corticosteroids		
Highly responsive	Psoriasis (intertriginous) Atopic dermatitis (children) Seborrheic dermatitis Intertrigo	Class 5, 6, 7
Moderately responsive	Psoriasis Atopic dermatitis (adults) Nummular eczema Primary irritant dermatitis Papular urticaria Parapsoriasis Lichen simplex chronicus	Class 3, 4, 5
Least responsive	Palma-plantar psoriasis Psoriasis of nails Dyshidrotic eczema Lupus erythematosus Pemphigus Lichen planus Granuloma annulare Necrobiosis lipoidica diabeticorum Sarcoidosis Allergic contact dermatitis, acute phase Insect bites	Class 1, 2

keratotic or lichenified dermatoses and for disease of the palms and soles (Table A2).

Bibliography

1. Brazzini B, Pimpinelli N. New and established corticosteroids in dermatology. Am J Clin Dermatol 3:47, 2002 [PMID: 11817968].

2. Biola A, Ballardy M. Mode of action of glucocorticoids. Presse Med 29:215, 2000 [PMID: 10705903].

3. De Bosscher K, Vanden Berghe W, Haegeman G. Mechanism of anti-inflammatory action of immunosuppression by glucocorticoids: Negative interference of activated glucocorticoid receptor with transcription factors. J Neuroimmunol 109: 16, 2000.

ORAL STEROIDS

Of all the numerous oral steroids listed in Table A3, it must be noted that the long-acting steroids have persistent immuno-suppression and as a consequence have more side effects. The short-acting drugs are useful for emergencies like anaphylaxis. The ideal drug that can be used orally are the intermediate-acting steroids, which include prednisolone and deflazacort. The use of long-acting steroids is restricted to situations where immunosuppression is required.

Genomic effects are mediated by cytosolic receptors that alter expression of specific genes whereas non-genomic effects are mediated by steroid selective membrane receptors. Prednisolone and methylpredni-solone have similar genomic potency, but in high dose therapy, the non-specific non-genomic effect of methylprednisolone is more than threefold stronger. This is the reason for the empirical clinical preference for methylprednisolone for pulse therapy. For conventional oral therapy, deflacort and prednisolone are safe steroids to use, as they are short acting, which largely determines the side effects.

So far as oral use is concerned, there is no strong evidence to suggest that methylpre-dnisolone confers any advantage over cheaper prednisolone. It is noteworthy that betamethasone has very low non-genomic potency because of which this drug is rarely used systemically although it has the same genomic potency as dexamethasone. Thus, if a long-acting steroid has to be given, dexamethasone is the preferred drug.

General Principles of Systemic Steroid Therapy

- Assess the indications, risks, benefits, alternatives, and possible adjuvant thera-pies.
- Evaluate possible contraindications and side effects, with special attention to any past history of psychiatric illness, osteo-porosis, diabetes mellitus, glaucoma, hypertension, and peptic ulcer disease (Table A4).
- Corticosteroids are relatively contra-indicated in psoriasis, in which their withdrawal may incite a generalized pustular flare, and in atopic dermatitis, in which withdrawal may be extremely difficult and may be accompanied by exacerbation.
- Diagnose and treat any secondary infec-tion (such as impetigo, cellulitis, or erysi-pelas) before starting steroids. Also, a protein-purified derivative (PPD) should be planned at the start of a long course of glucocorticoid therapy. It takes an average

Table A3: Overview of systemic steroids					
Short acting	Equivalent dose (mg)	Glucocorticoid potency	Mineralocorticoid potency	Plasma half-life (min)	Biological half-life (hours)
Cortisone	25	0.8	0.8	90	8–12
Hydrocortisone	20	1	1	30	8–12
Deflazacort	6–9	5	0.5	120	<12 hrs
Prednisolone	4	5	0.5	200	12–36
Methylprednisolone	4	5	0.6	180	12–36
Triamcinolone	4	5	0	300	12–36
Dexamethasone	0.75	20–30	0	200	36–54
Betamethasone	0.6–0.75	20–30	0	200	36–54

Table A4: Contraindications to oral steroid therapy	
Absolute	Ocular herpes simplex Untreated tuberculosis
Relative	Acute or chronic infections Pregnancy Diabetes mellitus Hypertension Peptic ulcer Osteoporosis Psychotic tendencies Renal insufficiency CHF (excluding that secondary to active rheumatic carditis) Diverticulitis Recent intestinal anastomoses

of 12 days for a patient to become anergic after starting glucocorticoids, so there is adequate time to discontinue steroid therapy and to start isoniazid, if indicated.

- Monitoring: While they are on corticosteroid treatment, patients should be monitored, at least monthly, for the presence of any adverse reactions. Development of symptoms such as polyuria, polydypsia, abdominal pain, fever, or joint pain should be assessed. Blood pressure and weight as well as fasting blood sugar, complete blood count (CBC), and lipid and electrolyte levels should also be followed. In addition, a stool hemoccult and eye examination should be checked biannually.
- If acute infection, trauma, or surgery occurs during treatment, the steroid dose must be increased appropriately. Patients exposed to acute stress are at increased risk of adrenal crisis. Symptoms of adrenal suppression include weakness, lethargy, nausea, anorexia, fever, orthostatic hypotension, hypoglycemia, and weight loss.
- HPA axis suppression must be considered after short courses. The degree of suppression depends on the patient, dosage (including frequency and amount), duration, and route of treatment. Longer courses and divided doses increase the risk for complications. Pituitary-adrenal reserve in response to stress may be diminished for as long as 5 days after a 5-day course of 25 mg PO b.i.d. A single injection of triamcinolone acetonide may suppress adrenal responsiveness for 2 to 3 weeks or more. Patients should be informed of this potential risk.

- In most instances, the best route of administration is oral, and the drug of choice is prednisolone, which is short acting and inexpensive.
- Other routes of administration include intralesional, intramuscular, or intravenous. Intralesional corticosteroids allow concentrated delivery directly into the involved area with minimal risk of HPA axis suppression. Intramuscular injection is used less frequently owing to prolonged suppression of the HPA axis and inconsistent absorption. Intravenous corticosteroids may be used in stressful situations in patients already on long-term oral steroids.
- Although prednisolone is not teratogenic, there is some risk of adrenal suppression and growth suppression in infants exposed in utero or through breastfeeding.
- To prevent glucocorticoid-induced osteoporosis, the American College of Rheumatology guidelines recommend bisphosphonate therapy for all patients beginning long-term prednisolone at a dose >5 mg/day.

Dosage

To achieve maximal therapeutic benefit, systemic corticosteroids must be given in adequate dosage for a sufficient length of time. It is also desirable to commence treatment as early as possible in the course of the illness.

Alternate day therapy starting at double the daily dose must be considered when use for>1 month is necessary. The initial dose of prednisolone for an adult with conditions such as allergic contact dermatitis should be at least 60 mg daily. The course should be for 2 to 3 weeks. If the dose is too small or duration of treatment too short, a rebound phenomenon with generalized exacerbation of the rash and symptoms can occur.

A. Prednisolone

Prednisolone should be given as a single daily dose (before 8:00 a.m.) to minimize suppression of the normal diurnal cortisol secretions. Occasionally, split doses are needed early on in a disease to achieve adequate therapeutic control; once achieved, conversion to an every morning or every other day schedule as soon as possible is recommended. Low doses of prednisolone (2.5 to 5.0 mg) at bedtime have been used to maximize adrenal suppression in cases of acne or hirsutism of adrenal origin.

Suggested regimens for acute dermatoses are given below.

Preferred Methods

- Prednisolone 60 mg PO each morning for 5 days, 40 mg PO each morning for 5 days, 20 mg PO each morning for 5 days, then discontinue. This is the easiest and least expensive regimen.
- Prednisolone 60 mg PO each morning for 7 days, followed by prednisolone 30 mg PO each morning for 7 days.

Other Schedules

- Prednisolone 60 mg PO each morning for 3 days, 50 mg PO each morning for 3 days, 40 mg PO each morning for 3 days, and then taper by 5 mg/day to 0.
- Prednisolone starting with 60 mg PO the first day and decreasing by 5 mg. The total amount and duration of treatment may be varied.

B. Short-Acting Steroid (Deflazacort)

Deflazacort is a glucocorticoid derived from prednisolone. Clinical studies have indicated that the average potency ratio of deflazacort to prednisolone is 0.69–0.89 and 6 mg of deflazacort is equivalent to 5 mg of prednisolone. However, the therapeutic dosage ratio has been reported to range from 1:1.2 to 1:1.5.

6 mg of deflazacort has approximately the same anti-inflammatory potency as 5 mg prednisolone or prednisolone. Doses of deflazacort usually lie in the range 0.25–1.5 mg/kg/day.

Abrupt withdrawal of doses up to **48 mg** daily of deflazacort or equivalent for **3 weeks** is unlikely to lead to clinically relevant HPA-axis suppression in the majority of patients. In the following patient groups, gradual withdrawal of systemic corticosteroid therapy should be considered even after courses lasting for 3 weeks or less:

- Patients who have had repeated courses of systemic corticosteroids, particularly if taken for greater than 3 weeks.
- When a short course has been prescribed within one year of cessation of long-term therapy (months or years).
  - Patients who may have reasons for adrenocortical insufficiency other than exogenous corticosteroid therapy.
  - Patients receiving doses of systemic corticosteroid greater than 48 mg daily of deflazacort (or equivalent).
  - Patients repeatedly taking doses in the evening.

C. Long-Acting Steroid (Oral Mini-Pulse—OMP)

OMP refers to giving a higher than the usual daily dose of corticosteroid on two consecutive days a week and leaving the remaining five days treatment-free. A long-acting corticosteroid is preferred so that the effect lasts for about 3 days at a time. Hence, it is preferred to give a long-acting corticosteroid on two consecutive days in a week rather than once in three days to give the hypothalamic–pituitary–adrenal axis (HPA axis) time to revert back to normal before the next dose. The standard regimen is to give oral betamethasone 5 mg (5 of the 1 mg betamethasone tablets) after breakfast on Saturday and Sunday (or any other two consecutive days) every week. But it is better to give dexamethasone pulse which has been used in doses of 5 mg or 10 mg as betamethasone has little non-genomic effect.

D. Injectable Glucocorticoids

Time noted is the duration of their ability to suppress inflammatory reaction.
- Short acting (hours to days):
  - Dexamethasone sodium phosphate
  - Methylprednisolone
- Intermediate acting (1 to 2 weeks):
  - Betamethasone acetate
  - Betamethasone sodium phosphate
  - Dexamethasone acetate
  - Triamcinolone diacetate
- Long acting (3 to 4 weeks):
  - Triamcinolone acetonide
  - Triamcinolone hexacetonide

The most commonly used steroid is triamcinolone acetonide and the concentration depends on the site of injection and the nature of the lesion. Lower concentrations (2 to 3 mg/mL) are used on the face to prevent atrophy of the skin, whereas keloids may require concentrations of 40 mg/mL. It is best to limit the total monthly dose of triamcinolone acetonide to 20 mg to ensure that the hypothalamic–pituitary–adrenal axis is not suppressed. There are serious drawbacks to intramuscular administration because of erratic absorption and lack of daily control of the dose. Because triamci-

nolone acetonide is longer acting than prednisolone, there are more potential side effects, including increased hypothalamic pituitary adrenal (HPA) suppression and myopathy.

Methylprednisolone is used in a dose of 500 mg to 1 g daily because of its high potency and low sodium-retaining activity. Serious side effects associated with intravenous administration include anaphylactic reactions, seizures, arrhythmias, and sudden death. Other adverse reactions include hypotension, hypertension hyperglycemia, electrolyte shifts, and acute psychosis. Slower administration over 2 to 3 hours has minimized many of the serious side effects, and as long as vital signs are determined frequently, patients without underlying renal or cardiac disease do not need to be monitored. It is important though to monitor serum electrolytes before and after pulse therapy, particularly when patients are on concomitant diuretic therapy. Recent studies suggest that doses that are less than the traditional high-dose (1 g methylprednisolone daily for 3 days) IV pulse therapy may be equally efficacious and safer.

Tapering Schedule of Oral Steroids

1. The daily dose is first gradually tapered to 40 or 50 mg of prednisolone.
2. Either the dose can be kept constant on 1 day and reduced on the alternate day by 5 mg decrements down to 5 mg/day, or, the steroid dose can be increased on 1 day and reduced by a similar amount on the alternate day.
3. After dose is tapered to 5 mg on alternate days, the 8 AM plasma cortisol level is measured 4 weeks after the 5 mg dose has been reached. If the plasma cortisol level is less than 10 mg/dL, the alternate day prednisolone dose should be decreased by 1 mg every 1 to 2 weeks to a maintenance dose of 2 mg/day. Then the 8 AM plasma

cortisol level should be rechecked every 2 months until it is greater than 10 g/dL, at which point maintenance GCs can be terminated.

4. Recovery of the HPA axis can take longer than 9 months. The HPA axis is rapidly suppressed after the onset of GC therapy. However, if therapy is limited to 1 to 3 weeks, the recovery of the HPA axis is rapid. Longer daily GC therapy is associated with suppression of the HPA axis for up to 1 year after therapy is terminated.

5. During any stressful situations, it is necessary to give high doses of GCs, generally 25 to 70 mg/day of prednisolone or 100 to 300 mg/day of cortisol in divided doses. Thus 25 mg of hydrocortisone equivalents for minor surgeries, 50 to 75 mg for moderate surgeries, and 100 to 150 mg for major surgery for 2 to 3 days, is advisable to patients who have been given long durations of steroids.

Special Monitoring and Advice

Diet

Diet should be low in calories, fat and sodium, and high in protein potassium and calcium. Protein intake is important to reduce steroid-induced nitrogen wasting. Use of alcohol, coffee and nicotine should be minimized. Exercise should be encouraged.

Infections

Patients with a positive PPD should be given prophylaxis with isoniazid. Some advocate use of Bactrim prophylaxis (1 DS Bactrim 3 days a week) against *Pneumocystic carinii* when patients receive concomitant cytotoxic therapy.

Gastrointestinal Complications

Although there is controversy about whether an increase in the incidence of peptic ulcer disease occurs in otherwise unaffected patients receiving GCs, there is almost a ninefold increase in patients taking both GCs and nonsteroidal anti-inflammatory agents.

Adrenal Suppression

Patients receiving daily GC therapy for longer than 3 to 4 weeks must be assumed to have adrenal suppression that requires tapering of the GCs to allow for recovery of the HPA axis. Tapering is best performed by switching from a single daily dose to alternate day doses, followed by a gradual reduction of the amount of the drug (*see* above).

An overview of monitoring is given in Table A5.

Steroids in Pediatric Population

In the pediatric population, GCs cause growth retardation and early osteoporosis. Growth retardation is not necessarily prevented by alternate day GC regimens. Immunization with live vaccines can be done, if the duration of GC use is less than 2 weeks at any dose, if the dose of GC is less than 2 mg/kg or 20 mg/day of any duration and if long-term alternate day treatment with short-acting preparations is done.

Complications

Complications associated with systemic GC therapy increase with higher doses, longer duration of therapy, and more frequent administration. However, osteoporosis and cataracts develop with alternate day dosing, and avascular necrosis (AVN) can be seen after only short courses of GCs. Though a list is given in Table A6, we will focus on the common problems.

Osteoporosis

Osteoporosis occurs in 40% of individuals treated with systemic GCs; it is especially prominent in children, adolescents, and postmenopausal women.

1. Approximately 30% of patients have evidence of vertebral fractures after 5 to

Table A5: Prevention of side effects with chronic (3 months) glucocorticoid use

Symptoms	Management
Hypertension	Blood pressure (baseline; repeat with each visit)
Weight gain	Weight (baseline; repeat with each visit)
Re-activation of infection	Purified protein derivative, anergy panel at baseline (can be done up to 12 days after starting prednisolone)
	Hepatitis screen
	Consider pneumocystis carinii pneumonia prophylaxis (Bactrim 1 DS three times a week)
Metabolic abnormalities	Electrolytes, lipids, glucose [baseline; repeat early after starting therapy; repeat annually; more frequent monitoring with known factors (e.g. diabetes, hyperlipidemias)]
Osteoporosis	Bone density (baseline; repeat annually, if early bone prophylaxis done). Instruct about diet, exercise, other measures
	Calcium and vitamin D supplementation
	Start bisphosphonate for men, postmenopausal women.
	Evaluate postmenopausal women for hormone replacement therapy.
	Serum testosterone after treatment started in men; if low (<300 ng/mL), check prostate-specific antigen, prostate examination before starting testosterone replacement.
Eyes	Cataracts: Slit-lamp examination (every 6–12 months).
	Glaucoma: Intraocular pressure examination (at 1 month and every 6 months).
Peptic ulceration	In patients with two or more risk factors, consider prophylaxis with H_2-antagonist or proton pump inhibitor.
Suppression of hypothalamic–pituitary–adrenal axis	Single, early morning doses, preferably every other day. Check 8 AM serum cortisol before tapering prednisolone <3 mg/day. If <10 g/dL, repeat every 1–2 months and maintain low prednisolone dose until baseline cortisol adequate.

10 years of GC treatment, but this proportion is higher in postmenopausal women.

2. Bone loss occurs most rapidly in the first 6 months of GC use, but continues at a slower rate after that, with loss of 3 to 10% of bone per year in many patients.

3. Low doses of prednisolone (2.5 mg/day) adversely affect bone and increase vertebral and hip fractures.

Trabecular bone is primarily affected, leading to painful vertebral fractures.

Management of Complications

A list of common complication and methods to avoid them is given in Table A5 and A6. We will focus on the major complications here.

Osteoporosis

Calcium and vitamin D together, but not calcium alone, preserve bone mass in patients receiving long-term treatment with GCs at an average of 15 mg/day.

Table A.6: Common complication with systemic steroids	
Dermatologic	Acne Alteration of fat distribution (cushingoid appearance) Urticaria Facial erythema Atrophy Striae Lanugo hair Alopecia
Central nervous system	Pseudotumor cerebri Psychiatric disorders
Musculoskeletal Ocular	Osteoporosis with spontaneous fractures Aseptic necrosis of bone Myopathy Glaucoma Cataracts
Gastrointestinal	Fatty infiltration of the liver Nausea, vomiting Intestinal perforation Pancreatitis Peptic ulceration
Cardiovascular and fluid retention	Hypertension Sodium and fluid retention Hypokalemic alkalosis Atherosclerosis
Suppression of host defenses	Immunosuppression, anergy Effects on phagocyte kinetics and function Increased incidence of infections Recurrent tuberculosis
Endocrinologic	Suppression of hypothalamic–pituitary–adrenal axis Growth failure Secondary amenorrhea
Metabolic	Hyperglycemia Nonketotic hyperosmolar states Hyperlipidemia Drug interactions Fibroblast inhibition Inhibition of wound healing Subcutaneous atrophy (striae, purpura)

Patients taking GCs should be given elemental calcium, 1500 mg/day, and vitamin D, 400 units twice daily. Activated forms (alfacalcidiol 1g/day, or calcitriol, 0.5 to 1.0 g/day) can be given, but more frequent monitoring is required for hypercalciuria and hypercalcemia. Patients with a history of renal stones should not receive supplemental calcium and vitamin D.

Premenopausal women who become amenorrheic because of GCs benefit from hormone replacement therapy (HRT). Such therapy helps to prevent the effects of GCs on bone. For postmenopausal women; HRT is effective for preventing osteoporosis. The Women's Health Initiative, a large randomized controlled primary prevention trial, demonstrated that combined estrogen plus progestin significantly reduced fractures at the hip, vertebrae, and other sites compared to placebo. Postmenopausal women can be treated with oral conjugated estrogen (premarin), 0.625 mg/day. Women with a uterus should also receive medroxyprogesterone (provera), 2.5 mg/day, which prevents the increased endometrial carcinoma that occurs in women receiving estrogen alone.

Men with low serum testosterone levels who are receiving GCs should have testosterone supplementation. Based on recommendations published by the American Association of Clinical Endocrinologists and the American College of Endocrinology, men with serum testosterone levels below the physiologic range (less than 300 ng/mL) should receive replacement therapy. Testosterone replacement therapy can be considered, if a patient has a normal prostate-specific antigen test, and benign findings on prostate examination. Replacement is administered either by the intramuscular route (testosterone enanthate or cypionate, 200 mg intramuscularly every 2 weeks or 100 mg every week to avoid cycling) or by testosterone patches (4 or 6 mg applied daily). Serum testosterone should be checked after replacement to assure adequate treatment.

The increased osteolysis caused by steroids has led to the use of a number of agents that inhibit bone resorption, such as the bisphosphonates and calcitonin. As bone formation proceeds at a much slower pace than resorption, anti-resorptive drugs produce a period of time up to 2 years where formation is greater than resorption. Several intravenous and oral bisphosphonates are now available and have revolutionized the approach to prevention and treatment of steroid-induced osteoporosis. Oral bisphos-

phonates include alendronate, 70 mg/week or 5 mg/day (10 mg/day for postmenopausal women not on HRT); risedronate, 30 mg/week or 5 mg day; etidronate, 400 mg/day for 2 weeks every 13 weeks; and ibandronate, 150 mg/month. An overview of managing steroid-induced osteoporosis is given in Table A7 and Flowchart A1.

Atherosclerosis

Blood pressure, serum lipids, and glucose levels should be measured serially. Abnormalities should be treated with dietary manipulation and medication as necessary. Patients who smoke should be encouraged to stop. Female sex hormones protect against the development of atherosclerosis, and thus hormone replacement therapy for postmenopausal women on GCs makes sense. However, recent data suggest that women with established atherosclerosis actually do worse with hormone replacement therapy, and there was a 58% increase in coronary heart disease events in the first year after myocardial infarction in patients treated with an estrogen/progestin combination. If patients develop increased levels of cholesterol or triglycerides while taking GCs, there are now good approaches to treatment, particularly with some of the newer statins, that have impact on the development of atherosclerosis and prevent myocardial infarctions.

Patients should be treated or referred for treatment on the basis of guidelines that emphasize the importance of assessing the risk of atherosclerosis. These guidelines recommend treatment when patients have low-density lipoprotein (LDL) cholesterol levels greater than 160 mg/dL and fewer than two coronary heart disease risk factors (high LDL cholesterol, smoking, hypertension, diabetes, male sex, family history of premature heart disease), LDL cholesterol levels greater than 130 mg/dL with two or

Table A7: Prevention of osteopororis on steroids (GIOP guidelines)	
Prevention	Patients starting GC therapy at a dose equivalent to prednisolone >5 mg/day for 3 months or longer should. • Modify risk factors for osteoporosis (stop smoking, decrease excessive alcohol consumption) • Start regular weight-bearing physical exercise • Initiate intake of calcium (total 1500 mg/day) and vitamin D (400–800 IU/day) • Consider bone mineral density (BMD) testing to predict risk of fracture and bone loss • Initiate bisphosphonate therapy (alendronate 5 mg/day or 35 mg/wk, or risedronate 5 mg/day or 35 mg/wk).
Treatment	Patients on long-term GC therapy should be tested for osteoporosis using BMD measurement. If the T-score is <–1, consider: 1. Risk factor modification including reducing risk of falls 2. Regular weight-bearing physical exercises 3. Calcium and vitamin D supplementation 4. Replacement of gonadal steroids, if deficient 5. Bisphosphonate therapy (alendronate 10 mg/day or 70 mg/wk, or risedronate 5 mg/day or 35 mg/wk) If bisphosphonates are contraindicated or not tolerated, consider calcitonin as second-line agent, intravenous bisphosphonate (pamidronate or zolendronate), or parathyroid hormone Repeat BMD measurement annually or biannually

Flowchart A1: Approach to premenopausal women and men aged 50 years initiating or receiving glucocorticoid therapy (American College of Rheumatology 2010 Recommendations for the Prevention and Treatment of Glucocorticoid-Induced Osteoporosis)

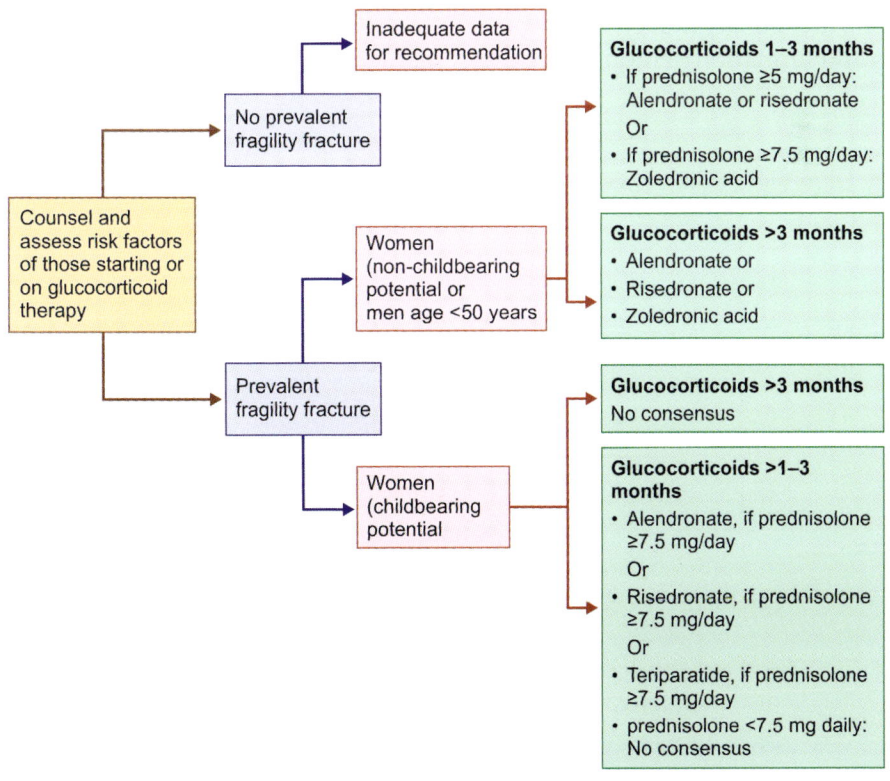

more additional risk factors for heart disease, and LDL cholesterol levels greater than 100 mg/dL for patients with established coronary artery disease. High-density lipoprotein cholesterol levels lower than 35 mg/dL independently predict increased coronary mortality rates in men and should be taken into account in therapeutic decisions. Several trials have demonstrated reduction in both coronary heart disease and total mortality rates with statin therapy. Patients should supplement the diet with folate and vitamin B_6 to control any elevations in homocysteine.

Avascular Necrosis (AVN)

Early detection is important because early intervention may prevent progression to degenerative joint disease requiring joint replacement. Twenty percent of patients with AVN have normal X-rays. Bone scan and magnetic resonance imaging are more sensitive techniques for evaluating AVN. Patients should be regularly questioned about pain and limitation of motion of joints.

If abnormalities develop, an X-ray, bone scan, or magnetic resonance imaging should be ordered. If imaging shows AVN, an orthopedic surgeon skilled in early intervention with core decompression may be able to halt progression of the disease. Patients with AVN have an increased risk that other joints will be affected. The progression of AVN to destructive joint disease may require joint replacement surgery.

Conclusion

Though oral steroids are possibly the most commonly prescribed drug, clinician rarely monitors the therapy. The chapter may seem to be comprehensive and complex but it is essential for any clinician using this drug to learn three aspects, monitoring, and prevention of osteoporosis and the art of tapering down steroids. It must be appreciated that in today's "medicolegal" times, prevention of side effects achieves a lot more than just ethical practice. If this can be achieved, the goal of this section is achieved.

Index